THE DELICIOUS QUICK-TRIM DIET

THE
DELICIOUS
QUICK-TRIM
DIET

SAMM SINCLAIR BAKER
& SYLVIA SCHUR

VILLARD BOOKS   NEW YORK

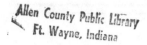
Library of Congress Cataloging in Publication Data

Baker, Samm Sinclair.
  The delicious quick-trim diet.

  1. Low-calorie diet. I. Schur, Sylvia. II. Title.
RM222.2.B345 1983 613.2'5   83–48074
ISBN 0–394–53431–X

Manufactured in the United States of America

9 8 7 6 5 4 3 2

First Edition

Designed by Oksana Kushnir

2213893

Contents

xi

1

WHY D.D. WILL WORK FOR YOU AS NO DIET EVER BEFORE

1

This One-Word Difference Means Weight-Loss Success and Lifelong _____Slimness at Last

At a dinner party the talk turned to diet, and a lovely, chubby woman sighed, "What the world needs is a diet that's pleasant, demands no real sacrifices, reduces you fast—and everything tastes perfectly delicious."

This is it—The Delicious Quick-Trim Diet ("D.D.").

D.D. works for you—bringing to life that one all-important word that represents a decisive difference between Quick-Trim reducing and any other weight-loss program: *Delicious.* D.D. cuts the calories but not the taste. For the first time, you'll enjoy speedy weight loss through Delicious, nutritious eating.

You'll lose up to a pound or more a day without feeling that you're sacrificing. You can stay beautifully trim for the rest of your potentially healthier, happier life—no matter how often you may have failed before.

And, so important to you, *D.D.'s clear, simple guidelines are in accord with findings in the landmark National Academy of Sciences report on diet, nutrition, and cancer.* You will be eating a proved, up-to-the-minute, nutritious balance of protein/fat/carbohydrates in delicious combination.

More good news from a national report: "Meeting in Boston under the auspices of the Harvard Medical School recently, the doctors affirmed the overall cancer-prevention value of a well-balanced, low-fat diet." They recommended percentages of 16% protein, 20% fat, 64% carbohydrates, which are close to the D.D. percentages chart in Chapter 4. D.D. eating also checks favorably with Harvard recommendations for low-fat cooking, low-fat dairy

3

products, and food vitamins. The primary aim of The Delicious Quick-Trim Diet is to reduce you swiftly, surely, deliciously—and it's a wonderful bonus that this healthful eating helps to prevent cancer and many common ills.

By cutting calories but not taste, D.D. eliminates a prime hangup that has kept many people from losing weight and keeping it off because of the common complaint: "I can't stand dull, unsatisfying food." Instead you'll applaud: "I'm losing pounds and inches, looking better every day, through truly delicious eating." Finally, here is your practical, pleasurable, *personal* success diet for eating at home or out. D.D. is sound, dependable, *the healthful, no-gimmick diet.*

The Quick-Trim fact, losing up to a pound or more a day, is absolutely essential to success for most people. When you see your weight dropping on the scale day after day, that will give you confidence—the *built-in willpower you need.* Here's a typical case history:

Betty W., a short, oversize woman who weighed 135 pounds, set her desired goal at 120 pounds. She went on one of those s-l-o-w reducing diets. After two long weeks of sacrifice, she was down to 133 pounds, and gave up in disgust. She told us, "I lost in two weeks only two pounds, and the willpower to keep dieting."

Here's what happened when she went on the Delicious Quick-Trim Diet:

START OF D.D.	END OF 1ST WEEK	END OF 2ND WEEK

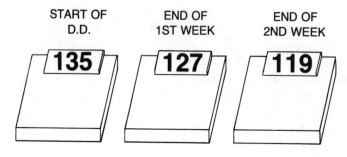

The scales tell the D.D. success story: She dropped from 135 pounds to 127 pounds in one week, and reported, "Nothing could stop me now—I'd lost eight pounds in one week, enjoying my meals, feeling great, and sacrificing nothing." In just one more week she'd reached her goal and surpassed it, was down to 119 pounds, looking beautifully slim. That was six months ago, and she's still a slim 120 pounds through D.D. Nutri-Maintenance Eating (see Chapter 15).

IMPROVES YOUR QUALITY OF LIFE

All important to you, the Delicious Quick-Trim Diet, plus lifelong D.D. Nutri-Maintenance Eating, improve in many *essential* ways on past weight-reduction methods. Delicious Dieting will help you get the most out of living, physically and emotionally. Our goal is to *enhance* rather than decrease your enjoyment of tasting and eating as you slim down and stay trim.

Another delighted, newly slim Delicious Dieter who took off 26 pounds and kept them off suggested, "You should call this the Quality of Life Diet, because delicious variety eating not only ends the usual drudgery of dieting, but also boosts thorough enjoyment of life."

Unique and realistic in its advances, D.D. erases once and for all the outmoded concept that rich, fatty, high-calorie food tastes best. You personally will discover—as excess pounds and inches vanish, and you feel so much healthier, look very much better—that now you can eat lean and love it. D.D. is also the first truly *personal* diet, designed for your individual tastes and choices: you select food according to your personal preferences, choosing what *you* want to eat. We believe that you'll make D.D. your way of eating always.

If you or someone in your household likes to cook, you'll be thrilled by the choice of easy, uncomplicated Delicious recipes to savor on the diet and afterward. You'll go for the dishes because of the superbly satisfying *taste*, beyond the low-calorie, low-fat slimming and health benefits. An excellent cook called these "the low-calorie servings with the high-calorie taste."

You'll soon appreciate the decisive difference between just eating, as most people do now, and knowing how to *taste* the D.D. way (Chapter 5). You'll get the most gratifying flavor and satisfaction from every calorie. The great French connoisseur, Brillat-Savarin, wrote: "He who eats too much knows not what to eat" and, we add, *how to taste*. You'll profit from the valuable new taste tips here.

So don't think of D.D. as just another weight-loss diet, but as an easy-to-learn course in tastier, more healthful eating and living from now on. No, you don't have to diet "forever" in order to stay trim. Once you're down to *your personal-choice desired weight*, and have learned the Delicious way of good eating, you can add many of the foods you prefer as an individual.

YOUR LICENSE TO INDULGE

Another wonderful, lifelong D.D. benefit: You'll have a license to indulge—to enjoy "forbidden" foods and drinks, once you're trim. You'll check your weight on the scale each morning, and the Five-Pound Switch Signal will help keep you from ever being overweight again. You'll have all the tools to shape your future beautifully, thanks to D.D.'s built-in special advantages in both the Delicious weight-loss and maintenance programs:

- *You'll enjoy your meals* instead of feeling deprived, dissatisfied, and therefore hungry. You'll get exceptional pleasure from true food flavors, and won't need oversalted, oversugared, overfatty dishes. In fact, you'll learn to reject them. As you see yourself losing up to a pound or more a day deliciously, you'll become increasingly confident of achieving slimness at last, and staying trim, as never before: You'll be saying, like others, "Great eating and results—I can keep going, no problem!"
- Without working at it consciously, you will acquire naturally, gradually, *a new way of tasting and eating* that keeps you from putting on excess pounds and inches again. No more "yo-yo" syndrome for you. The D.D. Nutri-Maintenance Balance of fine foods makes sense healthfully—no ineffective gimmicks such as "magical combinations," "enzyme miracles," "Spartan regimens." Life and food are meant to be enjoyed, not just endured.
- Choosing servings *you personally prefer* is another decisive advantage you'll appreciate, compared with other diets. You're a thinking individual, you can do it your way—and you'll love it! Feeling and looking your best eventually, enjoying food much more than before, you'll enhance your quality of life increasingly. And finally you'll be able to stay slim always, guided by that simple Five-Pound Switch Signal and lifelong Nutri-Maintenance Eating.

6

Summing up, the bottom line of why and how Delicious Quick-Trim eating will work for you at once and lifelong is simply this: *maximum good taste from every calorie—you eat deliciously, but you don't eat "fat."*

NOTE: We know that you are eager to start on the Delicious Quick-Trim Diet, and we're with you all the way—so you can begin trimming down immediately. You may wish to pause for a few minutes, perhaps to read Chapter 6 on the psychology supporting the exceptional effectiveness of Delicious Dieting—as further reassurance that at last you'll achieve the swift and lifelong slimming success you want so much.

2

Dual Experience Assures
Your Slimming
Success

We want to share this diet with you, Sylvia Schur and I, because we've proved that it works exceptionally, based on our long, successful experience with diet, nutrition, and food preparation. We have studied the effects of varied diets on millions of readers, and our new findings make for different, advanced guidelines—yours for the first time in this book.

I've enjoyed unparalleled success in helping people to reduce during more than twenty-five years of involvement in diet research and writing. The following blockbuster best sellers that I co-authored have helped reduce millions of overweights worldwide:

- *The Complete Scarsdale Medical Diet* (with Dr. Herman Tarnower), the best-selling diet book of all time. *The Doctor's Quick Weight-Loss Diet*, the number two best-selling diet book ever (with Dr. Irwin M. Stillman).
- *The Doctor's Quick Inches-Off Diet, The Doctor's Quick Weight-Loss Diet Cookbook, The Doctor's Quick Teenage Diet, Dr. Stillman's 14-Day Shape-Up Program* (all with Dr. Irwin M. Stillman).

Over 25 million copies of my diet books have been sold in all editions internationally.

I derived invaluable additional practical knowledge from countless contacts in person, and through loads of letters from overweights and successful dieters. All that, and working with

8

Dr. Tarnower and Dr. Stillman, plus my own extensive research through the years, has been incorporated with the most recent discoveries in the fields of diet and nutrition to produce *The Baker-Schur Delicious Quick-Trim Diet*. The result is a great advance in helping you to lose pounds and inches swiftly and healthfully, as never available before. The editor of a leading women's magazine told me, "This is the best diet book I've ever read!"

Most fortunately for all of us, I sought out and have been joined here in collaboration by the woman whom I (and many others) rate as one of the world's foremost experts in food and nutrition, and in food preparation. She has been called "the queen of good taste." Her experience and expertise now work for you in these pages.

Sylvia Schur has guided millions of readers to new, most tasteful diet and recipe discoveries. She established Creative Food Service over twenty years ago to serve the food interests of individuals, families, leading firms, and international agricultural producers.

In her own building and kitchens, she has assembled and directs a top-qualified group of food writers, cooks, researchers, and consultants. She has helped develop outstanding quality food products, reducing diets and recipes, and dozens of cookbooks on food preparation and serving.

Sylvia has been food editor of *Parade, Look, Woman's Home Companion, Seventeen*, and other major magazines, and now writes the respected newsletter, *Food Wise*. As America's leading food writer, she has written articles for *Family Circle, Woman's Day, House Beautiful*, and many other publications.

Every Delicious recipe in this book was tested in the Creative Food Service kitchens under Sylvia's supervision. That's your assurance that D.D. recipes are simple and easy to prepare, tops in quality, nutrition, and delicious taste—and affordable. The result for you from this expert partnership is a new, more delicious, and healthful way of eating to help you to slim down and stay trim, along with a new, better way to prepare and enjoy food.

Also important, this book has been checked by various experts, including a physician, Dr. Stanley M. Pearlman, two doctors of psychology, Dr. Ester R. Shapiro and Dr. Jeffrey Baker, and a doctor of science. You can be certain that you can now reduce and stay slim positively and Deliciously—and reach your goal of a healthier, happier lifetime.

3

How the Delicious Diet
Works for You
____Ten Basic Ways

1. It's SURE.

The Delicious Quick-Trim Diet cannot help but work for you—*if you will work with it*. The diet is constructed on specific proved weight-loss principles that have helped *hundreds of thousands* of overweight people to reduce with our personal experience and guidance. Distinctive, advanced new D.D. features help assure your quick and lasting weight loss. If you don't lose weight on this diet, you're not following instructions correctly.

2. It's SIMPLE.

You don't count calories (although calories *do* count). You don't weigh foods. You don't measure portions. You simply eat according to the daily listing for breakfast, lunch, and dinner each day. You have the all-important benefit of *enjoying* what you eat—your personal choice from seven breakfasts, lunches, and dinners. For example, you're not limited to Monday's chicken dinner, if you prefer Wednesday's casserole or Friday's fish on that particular day.

3. It's SENSIBLE.

With D.D., you can eat at regular family meals, attend lunch and dinner parties, dine in restaurants—without being restricted to specific foods to the point of feeling like a freak. If you like to cook, Delicious recipes are easy to prepare. You don't have to search out hard-to-find ingredients. Here, at last, are the *truly* "light" foods that, as *The New York Times* headlined, "are conquering America"—and, we add, the world.

4. It's SELECTIVE.

We must emphasize this feature of the Delicious Diet because arbitrary and unnecessary restrictions have kept many well-intentioned dieters from adhering to their diet, and therefore failing. You'll save money because, for instance, you can buy the food you want when it's on "special" at the store; you don't have to buy higher-priced "striped bass" because it's specified on your diet that day.

It makes sense that a restaurant gives you a *choice* from the menu listing. You don't have to settle for one take-it-or-leave-it offering. Similarly, on the Delicious Diet, you have alternates—you can choose from seven different mix-and-match breakfast, lunch, and dinner listings. No more "this is Tuesday, it must be turkey." Selectivity is just another practical reason why you will trim off pounds more quickly, surely, and steadily on this diet. And selectivity in the *quality* of foods you choose also will help you enjoy better flavors and new eating experiences.

5. It's SPEEDY.

You lose up to a pound or more a day, day after day—depending on how overweight you are. The heavier you are, the more quickly the excess pounds will come off, of course.

6. It's SUCCESSFUL.

If you're 10 pounds overweight, you can take it off in one to two weeks with Delicious Quick-Trim Dieting. No dragging along for months on a slow-reducing regime, where most people fail. Here's another typical result—in this case a woman five feet three inches tall who weighed 136 pounds and wanted to get down to 115 pounds:

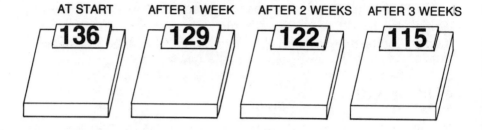

AT START	AFTER 1 WEEK	AFTER 2 WEEKS	AFTER 3 WEEKS
136	129	122	115

7. It's SAFE.

On the Delicious Basic Diet, your foods include poultry, fish, shellfish, cheeses, eggs (within limits), vegetables, fruits, breads, and other healthful, nutritious foods. This is not a one-dimensional diet, not a "gimmick" or "fad" diet.

8. It's SUSTAINING.

With this kind of Delicious variety eating, people find that they are never hungry, never tired—but happily satisfied. Without strain, you learn the light, lower-calorie, enjoyable way of eating that can keep you trimmer and healthier lifelong. You'll delight in the increasing reward of looking and feeling better. Simple instructions tell you how—the rest is up to you.

9. It's SUPPORTIVE.

Your self-image zooms from the first day you start the Delicious Diet. Look in the mirror daily, without clothes, after you step off the scale. You'll get a wonderful emotional lift as you see the pounds and inches melting away. Friends will say, "You're looking terrific!" But the most supportive boost is the self-knowledge that *you're* doing it, *you're* taking action to improve yourself. And the main, continuing motivation is that you see yourself and feel yourself trimming down *Deliciously*.

10. It's SUPER-DELICIOUS.

You'll learn a new way to *taste* and enjoy every mouthful as never before, a vital part of effective reducing and good living. Here you'll find not empty theory, but simple how to's that will work for you.

If you like to cook, you'll love the delectable, easy-to-prepare recipes and menu selections that give you a wide range of choice. If dinner specifies chicken, for instance, you select your preference from a dozen recipes such as D.D. Stir-Fry Vegetables with Chicken or Turkey, and D.D. Chicken Cacciatore (the light, luscious, lower-calorie Creative Food Service version of the famous Italian specialty).

Or—of course—prepare chicken your own favorite way, or eat the chicken offered in a restaurant—within the Delicious Diet specifications.

If fish and shellfish are listed, choose from D.D. Baked Flounder Florentine, D.D. Scallops in Green Sauce, and many more simple recipes. Or cook the fish and shellfish your own favorite way, or as offered in a restaurant—but always within Delicious Diet guidelines.

Family and guests, as well as you, will enjoy these D.D. super-Delicious servings with super-satisfying flavors. All are created to slim you surely and healthfully. *They'll work for you.*

4

The Scientific How: D.D. Nutri-Slimming Balance

The goal of this book is to help you lose weight, not to confound you with complicated scientific theory. We want what you want, to help you slim down and stay trim—period. That's what the Delicious Quick-Trim Diet will deliver.

You may wish to skip even this brief and necessarily simplified explanation of how D.D. works. Or . . . you may be one who is aided by a clearer understanding of the scientific principles behind D.D. If you want to know the *why* as well as the *how* of Delicious Dieting, here are some brief, basic facts that will illuminate why D.D. works so effectively.

No matter how much anyone tries to muddle the issue with sleight-of-mind promises of "miracles" in pseudoscientific terms, weight loss for the average adult in normal health is a matter of *calories-in, calories out*. If you consume more calories daily than your body uses up in function and activity, the excess calories are deposited as *pockets of fat* in your body.

The human body is a marvelous mechanism. The "fat pockets" provided for primitive men and women were a source of energy when they had to go without solids for days, even weeks, due to scarcity of meat, fish, and other foods. During periods of deprivation, the system pulled energy from the fat pockets—*the body feeding on itself*.

Today, basically, the functioning of the body is the same: When you consume more calories in food and drink than you use up in day-by-day activity, fat pockets are enlarged within you. When you pile in excess calories meal after meal, your body swells and bulges. Enlarged fat pockets crowd your organs, inhibiting most effective functioning.

Your heart, other internal organs, your spine, bones, legs, feet must support the excess *living* fat. The fat is *not* the dead white matter you see on raw meat. Each bit of fat is a living organism, requiring blood and life support. The more excess fat, the more effort is required by your heart and system.

To lose weight, you cut calorie intake below calorie expenditure—simple as that. The Delicious Quick-Trim Diet was created to add pleasure while you reduce your calorie intake healthfully and swiftly. D.D. provides an essential element missing from other diets: *Delicious, satisfying eating*.

The taste fulfillment and gratification you get on D.D. are crucially important in helping you to get down to your desired weight and to maintain it lifelong. You cut calories but not taste. You eat deliciously and nutritionally, as delineated in the following:

VITAL REDUCING FORMULA:
D.D. NUTRI-SLIMMING BALANCE

In order for your system to thrive and function best, the human body needs three basic sources of fuel supply for heat and energy: protein, fat, and carbohydrates (P-F-C). Volumes could be (and have been) written about P-F-C, telling you probably more than you need and care to know. Here are brief explanations of their primary roles:

PROTEIN, the most plentiful substance other than water in the body, encompasses a number of organic compounds that occur in all living plants. These have been called "building materials," and are essential for all life processes, growth, and development in humans, animals, and plants.

Proteins contain *amino acids* as their basic structural units, necessary to produce enzymes, antibodies, and cells—for the growth, repair, and maintenance of tissues. Amino acids, "the building blocks of protein," supply nitrogen essential to life.

The *enzymes* produced (various complex organic substances) are involved in regulating body processes, and are capable of providing chemical changes, as in digestion. The *antibodies* help

15

prevent and combat disease and infection, aiding in the immune response and in overcoming toxic effects.

It's important to note that not all the protein foods, only those with "complete protein" ("high-quality protein"), such as meat, poultry, fish, and some dairy products, contain all the essential amino acids. Most vegetables and fruits are incomplete-protein foods, but can be balanced to offer complete benefits and have other valuable substances. D.D. aims to provide *both* in desirable balance. Proteins contain about 4 calories per gram.

FATS are various soft, solid, or semisolid organic compounds, composed primarily of fatty acids and glycerol. They occur in human and animal tissue and are a concentrated source of energy, vital in many functions. Fats play a part in providing some body insulation, and in furnishing some protection for various organs.

Fats are certainly not "all bad," but excessive quantities in the diet result in abnormal weight gain and even obesity, slowing digestion and absorption of food, often resulting in recurrent and severe indigestion. Excess fat spurs and aggravates many ailments.

Some fat is beneficial in providing *linoleic acid*, a polyunsaturated fatty acid essential in the human diet. It is of specific nutritional importance because the body cannot manufacture it, so it must be supplied in the food you eat. Only a very small amount of linoleic acid is needed by the adult body—*a minute percentage of the total calories*. Sufficient linoleic acid is supplied in foods on the Delicious Diet.

Vegetable fats, including polyunsaturated oils and margarine, which contain "unsaturated" fats, are generally considered more desirable in the human diet than animal fats (including butter), which are "saturated" and usually solidify at normal room temperatures or lower (not true of relatively "saturated" coconut oil and olive oil). However, all oils and fats, including polyunsaturated types, are high in calories (about 100 to 125 calories or more per tablespoon, 9 calories per gram), and must be used sparingly when reducing.

CARBOHYDRATES are a class of organic compounds composed of carbon, hydrogen, and oxygen. They include starches, sugars, and cellulose (ratio is approximately 2 hydrogen to 1 oxygen). Carbohydrates are practically essential—the chief source of energy for body functioning and exertion. They aid in assimilation and digestion of other foods.

Consuming an *excess amount* of carbohydrate calories, however, leads to overweight, even though no more "fattening" than an overabundance of protein or fats (keep in mind that carbohydrate and protein are 4 calories per gram, about half those of fat). When your diet includes the too-common overindulgence in starchy and sweet foods, high in refined carbohydrates but low in vitamins, minerals, and cellulose, the result will probably be overweight and the possibility of deficiencies in vitamins and essential amino acids.

ACHIEVING THE NUTRI-SLIMMING BALANCE

The bottom line is that eating an *excess of calories* from any source produces overweight. That's why the Delicious Quick-Trim Diet is specifically limited in calories in the healthful, desirable D.D. Nutri-Slimming Balance—to help you reduce swiftly, safely, surely:

- You get enough of the building blocks of *protein*, but not an excess.
- You get sufficient *linoleic acid* to supply your body needs, without piling in excess fat calories.
- Your body gets plenty of *complex carbohydrates* from vegetables, fruits, and whole grains—differing from an overabundance of the *simple carbohydrates* in sugars.
- On D.D., you consume enough but not an excess of *fiber* or roughage to aid elimination and regularity, helpful too in providing a feeling of fullness. Fiber is derived from plant sources, consists of complex carbohydrates such as cellulose and other compounds that are part of the structural formations of plants. But beware: Too much fiber can be destructive!
- D.D. furnishes essential *vitamins* and *minerals* from the leafy vegetables, fruits, poultry, fish, eggs, cheese, and meats (the latter on the Delicious Quick-Trim Variety Diet). To supply average needs, D.D. eating includes iron, calcium, phosphorus, iodine, copper, magnesium, potassium, zinc, and other elements.

17

A NOTE OF CAUTION: Moderate amounts of vitamins and minerals (as supplied in balanced eating) are essential, and a reasonable daily vitamin-mineral supplement may be helpful, and is not likely to be harmful. But overdoses of some vitamins and minerals can sicken you and be dangerous

- D.D. is low in *cholesterol*, a fatty material existing to a greater or lesser extent in the blood. While a high blood cholesterol level is generally conceded as undesirable, ongoing research is necessary to pin down clear conclusions. Evidence indicates that while some cholesterol is appropriate in humans, too much is bad, increasing the dangers of coronary heart disease and stroke.
- D.D. is low in *salt* and *sugar* intake (see Guidelines later).

To make sure that your body receives the required nutrients, the healthful D.D. Nutri-Slimming Balance has been worked out in accord with our experience in helping *millions* of overweights worldwide to reduce. (Nevertheless, as cautioned repeatedly, you must be checked and guided fundamentally by your physician.) D.D. composition is moderately high in protein, very low in fat, and moderately low in carbohydrates, using primarily complex carbohydrates.

There is absolutely no need to measure out with slide-rule precision exactly how much P-F-C and vitamins, minerals, and other elements you're getting in every meal and in everything you eat. The portions indicated are designed to provide what you need.

The following charts show how the typical American diet, which has resulted in overweight for many, compares with the Delicious Quick-Trim Diet in daily intake of protein, fat, and carbohydrates. P-F-C bars are shown first in *percentages*, then in numbers of *calories*:

DAILY INTAKE IN PERCENTAGES
PROTEIN . . . FAT . . . CARBOHYDRATES

The *percentages* of P-F-C calories, comparing average daily intake in the typical American diet, are derived from government and medical sources. Note the very low percentage of protein eaten, when compared with high fat and carbohydrate intake. See how consumption on the Delicious Quick-Trim Diet increases protein, cuts fat about in half, increases carbohydrates moderately (primarily "complex")—in *percentages*. (The next chart shows what happens with *calorie* intake.)

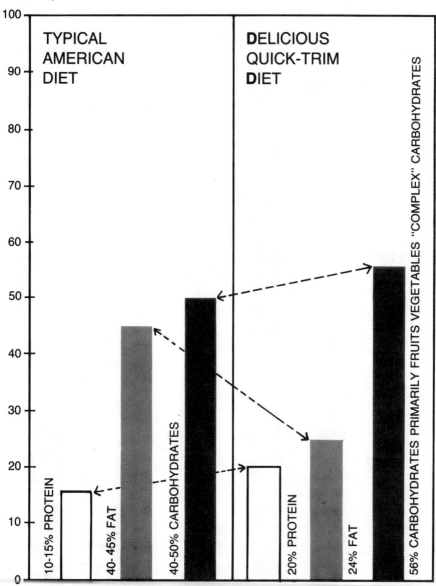

DAILY INTAKE IN CALORIES
PROTEIN . . . FAT . . . CARBOHYDRATES

Figuring a conservative 3,000 calories daily intake on the typical American diet (many overweights consume up to 5,000 and more calories daily), see what happens: With 1,000 calories average daily on D.D., high-protein calorie consumption is lowered. Fat calories are very low, but include essential linoleic acid. Carbohydrate calories are lowered substantially, are primarily "complex" carbohydrates from vegetables, fruits, and whole grains, not simple sugars.

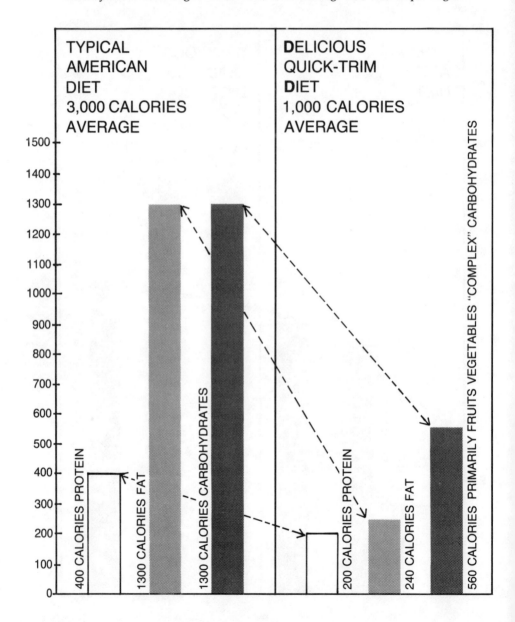

HOW YOU LOSE A POUND OR MORE DAILY

Summing up: On the Delicious Quick-Trim Diet, with its desirable nutritional balance, you follow the clear, simple guidelines in Chapter 9, and thus cut down to about 1,000 sustaining (and Delicious) calories per day. That's a big drop from the many more calories daily you have been consuming if you are overweight; your eating has probably been lopsided toward excess calories from fats and simple carbohydrates via sugars, sweets, and other high-calorie items.

Definitely, as an adult in normal health, you will lose up to a pound or more a day when you adhere to D.D. instructions—and you're assured by the exclusive D.D. benefit that you'll lose pounds and inches without losing the enjoyment of Delicious eating.

Realize, too, that consuming 1,000 calories daily on D.D. is not your "forever" course, but only until you get down to your desired weight. After that, you switch to D.D. Nutri-Maintenance Eating, as detailed in Chapter 15.

IMPORTANT NOTE ON LOSING "ONLY WATER"

It's common to hear uninformed, biased critics say, when someone loses weight rapidly on a diet, "She (he) is only losing water." The scientific fact is this:

When you decrease your calorie intake below calorie outgo and lose pounds, you lose fat and water. The value for calories expended only takes into consideration the *solids* in the fat cells. All body cells have a large proportion of water. When fat is lost from the body, the water contained in fat cells is thrown off. This water (which might be called "intracellular" water) has weight *that is not regained unless the fat is regained*.

If you gain weight, you add fat cells, thus add fat and water, and you put on pounds. If you don't put on more fat, you don't increase water weight either.

The solution: Take off the excess pounds swiftly on the Delicious Quick-Trim Diet. Don't add weight—and you won't add pounds and inches again. You'll stay trim with D.D. Nutri-Maintenance Eating. Watch the scale every morning; if you start gaining, you stop at the Five-Pound Switch Signal or before. Go back on D.D. for a few days, and you'll stay slim and trim—*and never be heavy again*.

21

5

How to Taste Deliciousness to Slim Down and Stay Trim

Here is a prime necessity, usually overlooked, to help you lose weight and keep it off: You must learn, as you will, finally, in this book and through the slimming D.D. daily menus, how to *taste* each bit of food you eat—versus just stuffing your mouth and swallowing, as so many overweight people do. You'll find that tasting *deliciousness* is one simple, sure way to improve your quality of life. And it doesn't cost more than the way you eat now, probably less.

Note this typical example of how many people eat without tasting: Our friend Adam, more than 30 pounds overweight, visited one night. He sat down next to a bowl filled with a pound of nuts. He talked—and munched. Suddenly his wife cried out, "Adam, you've finished the whole bowl of nuts yourself!"

He said, in shock, "My God, I didn't even know I was eating!"

When he learned on the Delicious Diet how to *taste* instead of just consume food, he lost weight rapidly—20 pounds in two weeks—and has kept it off ever since. He acknowledges that he'd never enjoyed eating as much as now, and he finds it easy to stay trim. We're certain that you'll say the same. You'll undoubtedly become a truer judge of taste in food, and probably in other matters that count. As Charles Lamb put it, "I hate a man who swallows his food affecting not to know what he is eating. I suspect his taste in higher matters."

Gourmets *taste* their food; gluttons gobble it and debase the food and themselves.

SIMPLE TECHNIQUES OF TASTING

Detailed instructions in tasting, eating better, and yet staying trim through the years will be covered in Section 3—after you have read Delicious Diet Guidelines, started dieting and losing weight rapidly. Here are some brief fundamentals to keep in mind with every meal you eat from now on:

1. *Look before you gobble:*　Take a tip from expert, caring wine tasters in approaching the taste of what you are about to eat. The connoisseur doesn't just hoist the glass and swig the wine in one insensitive gulp. The world's finest wine is tasteless if you don't take the time to appreciate it in every dimension. The same is true with food—eat with all your senses, and you won't just grab and cram it down.

2. *Examine colors and shapes:*　When did you last inspect with care the food you were about to eat? Did your *eyes* first appreciate the rich green of tender, perfectly cooked fresh asparagus? Recently we sat next to an obese individual in a superb restaurant and asked, "Aren't these long asparagus spears beautiful in shape and color?" He stared at his already emptied plate and mumbled, "I didn't notice"; he burped and added, "There weren't enough." He'd bolted them sightlessly without really enjoying them.

3. *Arrange your foods attractively:*　You'll find that there's far more satisfaction when you eat with your eyes too, not just with your mouth. With a little care, anyone can arrange on a dish a golden broiled fish fillet topped with a sparkling sprinkle of chopped chives, and bordered by a parade of glistening snow peas, orange spheres of firm cooked carrots, and sprigs of watercress. Here's a delight to eat, low in calories, high in eye and taste satisfaction— far more than mounds of rich, fattening foods dumped haphazardly on a plate.

4. *Enjoy the aroma:*　A true epicure wouldn't think of sipping a tawny Cognac without examining and admiring the color first, then swirling the liquid in the glass and inhaling the rich aroma. The full fragrance helps pleasure the taste immeasurably—and the same is true to get your utmost enjoyment from food.

5. *Taste the textures:*　To most appreciate what you're eating, you'll learn to test texture discriminately. Is it chewy? grainy? smooth? crusty? crisp? gummy? tender? tough? Once you give thoughtful attention to texture, you'll get greatest satisfaction from good food—and bypass servings that put on excess pounds without contributing to your eating pleasure.

23

6. Savor the flavor slowly: You've seen many overweights sweep a loaded plate clean when many others at the table have hardly begun to eat. Already that plump individual may be reaching for seconds. Ask how the food tasted and he's likely to say, with a troubled glance, "Okay, I guess." You'll find that less food, and fewer calories, are more satisfying to the taste when eaten slowly and appreciatively. Gobbling hurriedly is as wasteful (and unhealthy) as whizzing by a glorious scene in a car at 100 miles an hour.

7. Seek a balance of flavors: Many dishes, perhaps most, are oversalted, oversugared, and overfatty, to compensate for a lack of true, good flavors. Eating the D.D. way will bring you its own rewards in eating enjoyment, as well as in weight loss. Much overweight is due to *missing* real, gratifying flavor, therefore eating more and more—too much—in the search for taste gratification.

We'll bet that you're more discriminating than you know. If you race through a big portion of excessively oiled, heavily salted pasta with greasy meat sauce and still reach for more—your palate is probably searching for a true balance of flavors that the excesses of high-calorie ingredients don't provide.

You'll learn here how to prepare low-calorie, high-flavor foods at savings in calories and money, how to make the right selections at the market—and how to choose and specify more tasteful, more healthful, calorie-saving dishes when eating out.

ONLY FOUR BASIC FLAVORS

You may be surprised to find out that there are only four basic flavors: sweet, sour, salty, and bitter.

But ah, the variations you can play when you know how, just as you learn how to hear the notes in a song. You'll discover, for instance, that these four key flavors are tasted in different areas of the tongue. Because sour sensation comes next to salty on your tongue, a dash of lemon juice can often replace salt effectively.

You'll master the distinction between delicate, Delicious seasoning, and unhealthy overseasoning. A touch of salt, pepper, herbs, sugar, a score of seasonings, a little sweet butter, and other enhancing ingredients are used just right to improve flavors on the Delicious Diet.

You can train yourself, as taught here, how to discern ultimate desirable tastes, and to get the greatest eating enjoyment from them—without overeating. Once you know how to taste—*really taste*—you'll find that it's taste, not bulk, that satisfies the appetite most.

Then you'll make your motto for life: A little is as good as a feast when you really enjoy it—and *nonfattening*. Thoreau emphasized, "He who distinguishes the true savor of his food can never be a glutton; he who does not cannot be otherwise."

6

The Psychology Supporting Delicious Quick-Trim Dieting

For a diet program to work, it has to be psychologically sound. It has to have enough built-in incentives and rewards so you will stick with it throughout, confident of success—and then see it proved by wonderful results. D.D. provides exactly what you need and want, as not offered by any weight-loss program before.

Briefly, here are fundamental specifics of the psychology supporting D.D. methodology and benefits for you:

1. IMMEDIATE REWARD

From your first D.D. meal, you realize—probably with surprise and delight—that you're eating *Deliciously*, making none of the difficult sacrifices most dieters have come to expect. This is extremely important to overcome the initial sense of *feeling deprived* on a diet.

Feelings of deprivation often lie behind much overeating behavior in the first place—through the dynamic of *displacement*. Subconsciously one may say, "I'm being deprived of many things I want, so I'll compensate by eating"—tending to lead to overeating and weight gain.

However, on D.D. you realize at once that, "I'm *eating well*." D.D. works for you because it embodies a basic principle of behavioral learning—that one changes (here, from overeating to effective reducing) *if rewards follow in close association*.

Delicious Dieting eliminates the letdown experienced on other diets from giving up something important to you, that is, the enjoyment of eating. Instead, with D.D., you're not giving up anything but the excess pounds and inches you abhor. You heave a sigh of relief, and you relax, eager to proceed to your weight-loss goal—now reachable at last.

D.D. menus and recipes are varied, delectable, and satisfying by *experienced design*, to make every meal a treat rather than a sacrifice. Because what you are eating, which results in your losing weight swiftly, tastes good, you start acquiring at once a healthier psychology about dieting. You look forward eagerly to achieving your slim-trim goal, rather than dreading each dieting day, as in the past.

2. BUILT-IN WILLPOWER AND THE FEEDBACK PRINCIPLE

Built-in willpower is what you derive through the feedback principle, based on the *immediate weight-loss rewards* you can feel and see on your Delicious Diet—as contrasted with the failures of s-l-o-w dieting. Overweights who go on long-term diets designed to lose a pound or two a week tend to give up shortly with the common alibi, "I haven't the willpower to stick to the diet. I can't begin to see the light at the end of the tunnel." That's understandable. Even if it were desirable theoretically, the pound-a-week-loss diet simply *doesn't work* for most overweights.

Here's a specific example: A woman, Nancy T., who weighed 134 pounds and wanted to get down to 119 pounds, explained, "At the end of a week on a slow diet, I weighed 133 instead of 134 pounds—big deal. I looked ahead and realized that I'd have to stay on that bland, sacrificing diet for another three and a half *months* to get down to 119. I couldn't take it, so I quit, again feeling miserable, calling myself a weakling."

On the Delicious Quick-Trim Diet, she went from 134 pounds down to 127 within one week. She exulted, "I was gung-ho!" She started the second week by shifting to the Delicious One-Day Liquid Diet, then back to her Delicious Basic Diet for the rest of the week—and reached her goal, 119 pounds. "Beautiful!" She agreed that her "built-in willpower," based on the immediate feedback of watching the pounds come off, came spontaneously from stepping on the scale each morning to see her weight go down a pound a day—133 . . . 132 . . . 131 . . . and on down to her goal of 119 pounds within two weeks.

This lovely lady hadn't weighed under 120 pounds since her teenage years. Where there's D.D. built-in willpower, there's rapid weight loss—positively. You don't have to guess, you don't have to strive futilely for inner ego-strength, since you *know* that D.D. averages about 1,000 calories daily, yet satisfies deliciously. So by following instructions you *must* lose up to a pound or more a day.

---

3. EGO-STRENGTH SUPPORT

D.D. gives you support. You don't have to rely on yourself initially to make difficult or complicated decisions about what to eat at each meal every day, as on so many other diets that direct you to choose one from Column A, one from Column B, and so on.

With Delicious Dieting, you gradually take on the responsibility of choosing your menus to suit your personal tastes, but at the start you have specific, detailed support when you need it most. You let D.D. do the work of determining what you eat. No more bewilderment about "Decisions! Decisions! Decisions!" Gradually, as you slim down, you achieve the *self-mastery* that leads to enduring success in staying trim.

You avoid failure often due to supercilious "diet experts" who order, "Eat less." They know that most overweights became heavy in the first place because they have lost the ego-strength or willpower to control their consumption of food to "eat less."

Telling the stout person that her/his only way to reduce is to "eat less" is comparable to a lifeguard instructing a drowning person to "Swim!" That's correct, of course—swim and you won't drown. But the person is drowning because, unable to swim, she or he can't profit from the lifeguard's command.

Another parallel is a psychologist telling a patient to "stop being unhappy," or to "cut out" some self-defeating behavior that the person feels helpless to stop. If she could, she wouldn't have gone for professional help in the first place. Similarly, the overweight doesn't know how to "eat less"—so she fails, and keeps drowning in her own excesses.

She hasn't had the capacity, the ego-strength, to control her intake. So she's weighed down in every way, physically and emotionally in most cases, by the excess weight. The more she fails to "control herself," the more her self-esteem suffers, and the less *self-mastery* she experiences—and she probably continues to put on more unwanted pounds and inches. Thus she continues to ruin her appearance, her vigorous well-being, and her health—despite the admonition to "eat less." She hasn't been told and taught *how*.

Now, however, by instructing you precisely what to eat meal by meal, day by day, your Delicious Quick-Trim Diet states in effect: "I'm your ego-strength. Just follow the exact directions for what to eat. You can't help but lose up to a pound or more a day." That's the support you need. Follow the clear, simple guidelines comfortably—and you arrive at the slim, more attractive, free-moving body you seek—while also learning how to maintain your weight yourself.

The fact that you are told what to eat at each meal—with personal choices whenever you want to make them—makes Delicious Dieting a comparatively pleasant cinch, not a woe-is-me burden.

---

4. OBJECTIVE DAILY MONITOR

You don't *wonder* whether or not you are losing weight on your Delicious Diet—you *know* through this highly specific, *graphic* feedback: You step unclothed on the bathroom scale each morning upon arising, as instructed. You read and see the number on the scale and you know that you've lost another pound, that you're observing D.D. instructions correctly. Graphically you see the thrilling scoring of your success.

You record your weight on the Daily Scale Weight Chart scorecard previously provided for you. Knowing exactly where you stand daily, you take corrective action accordingly, if needed. In one of his hilarious columns, Art Buchwald complained to a friend, "I weighed myself this morning and my wife took my scale's word against mine." You can't bluff the scale, even if you stand on one foot like a stork, nor can you delude yourself. That's assuring, dependable daily reinforcement for you.

5. LIMITED TIME FRAME

If an overweight feels that in order to get down to her desired weight, she'll have to diet "forever," motivation and action may destruct even before she begins. Such negative psychology becomes a disabling state of mind that prevents many from ever slimming down, even when warned by the physician about serious ills and deterioration due to burdensome excess fat.

An unhealthy stonewall attitude is countered by D.D.'s rapid-reducing results. The dieter is assured that she can be trim within a limited time frame. After you've trimmed down, you enjoy D.D. Nutri-Maintenance Eating lifelong, confident that you can stay slim.

If stress or other factors in living put pressure on you to resort to previous bad habits of overeating, the Delicious Diet comes to your rescue. Through the Switch System, which you will have learned, you return to the daily dieting guidelines that *proved* to you that you could lose weight rapidly.

6. NO ENDURING GUILT FEELINGS
NO SELF-DEFEATING BEHAVIOR

We tell you repeatedly now and elsewhere that there's no need for self-recrimination if you slip off your Delicious Diet for a day or so—or even for a social weekend or vacation—and gain back some of your lost weight. *You simply go right back on D.D.* There's no point in feeling guilty or depressed, since you know that if you overeat one day, you have the simple means to compensate the next day.

Thus, realistically based confidence overcomes the tendency to the self-doubt and self-criticism that lead to giving up after a misstep or a discouraging note. Your instructed action is clear: Return to your Delicious Diet, perhaps beginning with the Delicious Three-Day Vegetable Diet or One-Day Liquid Diet. Your scale will tell you immediately that you're losing any regained weight swiftly once more. *Your scale tells you so.* That banishes any guilt feelings and self-defeating behavior—you're succeeding in slimming down beautifully again.

Don't let scaremongers convince you that losing and gaining up to 10 pounds over a period of time is terrible for you. Only your personal physician, knowing your individual condition, can make the correct judgment. For the average person in normal health, some seesawing in weight is to be expected, and is accommodated readily by nature. Your body isn't a steel-plated precision machine—you're human and variable, and thanks be for that.

Do your best—and if you slip off your diet and gain a few pounds, it's not an enduring tragedy or health crisis (unless you have a serious health problem, and should be on a doctor-regulated regimen, as warned repeatedly in these pages).

It's no big deal to indulge now and then. It's wasteful to weep and wail, accusing yourself of being "weak" or "spineless." Such self-defeating feelings could become an obsessive substitute for effective, positive action. You slipped, and you acknowledge it—*and then you get on to D.D. business at once!* Reread D.D. guidelines and as much of this book as you have time for, keeping foremost in mind that D.D. will take off regained pounds.

There's no such thing as failure on D.D., because you always have another chance. There are so many Delicious dishes here that dieting becomes easier and more satisfying each day, instead of harder. Persistence brings you the sure payoff—a more attractive figure, increased vigor, a healthier potential.

Your attitude, like ours, is positive on D.D., never negative. We're totally against self-humiliation. We're appalled by an ad in a mail-order catalog offering a battery-powered gadget to place in the refrigerator. When the door is opened, the device screams, "You'll be sorry, Fatty!" or other offensive putdowns. Such insults are humiliating and destructive. We do enough of this to ourselves without such "help."

An overweight friend, a dignified and successful officer in a large corporation, visited a well-known, very costly "reducing doctor," and went on his diet, which included drugs. He returned for weekly weigh-ins—but wasn't losing weight. On the fourth visit, the frustrated physician swore at him, belittled him mercilessly. The patient responded quietly, "I don't take foul abuse from anybody. What I've lost here is several hundred dollars but not a single pound."

The fault wasn't necessarily the doctor's, whose methods had succeeded with some patients, although certainly not all. But one thing was sure: his psychological approach was inexcusable. That can't possibly happen on Delicious Dieting, where your instructions are plainly printed, based on sound psychological principles, and designed to help you feel better about yourself.

7. ACCUMULATED BENEFITS:
REDUCED POUNDS, MORE DAILY REWARDS . . .

With D.D. recipes conceived by Sylvia Schur and her highly respected Creative Food Service staff, you are rewarded with a wide variety of taste treats in each day's eating, including wine, if you like. Each item has been prepared and tested for luscious taste and low calories under Sylvia's personal direction. With D.D. servings, you are rewarded by good taste without sacrifice, as you lose weight rapidly.

You benefit in self-confidence and pride as you near your goal. This helps you change what has been called "fat behavior," such as trying to please an insistent hostess by taking another helping even when you're full. Instead, your new self-respect bolsters you to respond, "No, thanks. I've enjoyed what I've eaten, but I set my limit and never exceed it, no matter how tempting the food is." You enjoy not only weight loss, but a wonderful new sense of mastery.

As soon as you are down to your desired weight goal, you move on to Nutri-Maintenance Eating, again with precise, simple, clear instructions for maintaining your trim, attractive figure. You are rewarded with a daily increase in calories adjusted to sustain your trimness according to your height and personal intake/outgo of calories. You eat and drink happily according to pleasurable, relaxed guidelines.

You are instructed specifically in the D.D. Activity Plan (Chapter 17) about adapting activities, exercise, and sports toward expending maximum calories healthfully and comfortably. The aim is to be limber, to improve vigor, circulation, and muscle tone, according to your personal likes and capacities. You are assured, psychologically as well as physically, that it's not necessary to become a "jock" or super athlete in order to keep trim. No overexertion, no pain, no excess pressure. Enjoy!

You reward yourself with a *bonus*—our D.D. Nutri-Maintenance Recipes, which include "a touch of" some higher-calorie ingredients, desserts, other servings—all light, healthful, but never too rich, fatty, heavy, or greasy. You enjoy this bonus of better,

32

nutritious, satisfying eating for life. After all, a celebration is in order!

---

8. LIFELONG SLIM-TRIM CONDITIONING

By the time you have reduced to your desired weight and moved on to the liberal D.D. Nutri-Maintenance Eating, you have been conditioned physically and psychologically—almost without realizing it—to *prefer* lighter, healthier, Delicious eating.

You will have discovered through this natural behavioral change that overly rich, fatty, and high-calorie servings are not only undesirable and bad for your health, attractiveness, and well-being—but also unpleasing and even unpalatable. You've come to single out nonfatty, nonsugary, nonrich edibles—consciously and unconsciously. You have conditioned yourself over the D.D. days and weeks not by thinking but by *doing*. You have taken off your unwanted excess weight, and your body (as well as your mind) is happy about it.

Physically you feel much better slim—buoyant, free from indigestion and other bodily ills due to overweight. You're psychologically conditioned now to stay trim because you look and feel much more attractive. You exult in the pride and pleasure arising from your personal accomplishment. *You* did it!

The psychological lift from having achieved your goal is most gratifying and sustaining. Explaining his personal outlook after reducing to trim, handsome proportions, opera star Placido Domingo said, "Is not aesthetic for the stomach to hang out in front." Then he added, about forsaking rich, heavy foods, "Such a little pleasure to give up for such a lot."

---

9. NEVER HEAVY AGAIN

Now you have the tools to stay slim, even if you put on up to five pounds through special circumstances, such as binges for social or other reasons. You are guarded and guided by your daily "reality testing" weigh-in on the scale, coupled with the D.D. Five-Pound Switch Signal. Any time the scale shows five pounds above your desired weight (if you ever permit that to happen), psychologically a clamorous alarm bell starts ringing in your head.

As a result, rather than "feeling bad," punishing yourself by giving up, you go right back on the Delicious Diet of your choice. You return to your desired weight.

A dieter once told me that she uses the full-length mirror as an additional scale to weigh the shape of her body with her eyes. That's a thought, but be wary that your eyes don't diminish or exaggerate your dimensions, since their view is entirely personal and subjective. The weight scale is trustworthy because the accurate numbers are measured mechanically, thereby impersonally. The scale tells the truth; it doesn't punish, as your subjective vision might.

Another incentive, and vital D.D. bonus, is the assurance that you're not bound to a limited choice of foods. You have a selection, according to your preference, of *four* Delicious Diets, each with simple, specific instructions that have been proved to reduce you rapidly, healthfully, Deliciously.

THE KEY: DO-IT-YOURSELF REALISM

You cannot help but lose weight if psychologically you accept the responsibility that dieting is do-it-yourself in order to succeed. The Delicious Quick-Trim Diet increases your chances for reducing successfully, as never before, because it provides the Deliciousness you want, along with the lower-calorie intake you need to lose weight. At the same time, it encourages and supports a *realism* that is good for you.

A typical example: I met a charming, plump woman at a dinner party. I found Anne bright and witty. She told me at one point, "I bought your latest diet book." I smiled and said, "Thanks." She went on, "Obviously I didn't lose any weight." I shrugged. "Too bad." After a pause, she touched my arm apologetically and said, "*I never went on the diet. . . .*"

Reading this book won't make you slim; going on the Delicious Diet will. Absorbing and adhering to D.D. Nutri-Maintenance Guidelines will keep you trim lifelong. Since you'll be eating an average of 1,000 calories per day or less, the pounds and inches will diminish. No excuses accepted about imbalanced metabolism or other systemic disorder—your doctor will have checked that and acted to correct the problem or given you special dietary advice.

Some overweight people blame society and media pressures for making them feel ashamed about being fat and trying to force them to be thin. They complain angrily that fashion magazines, fashion pages in newspapers, fashion tips on TV and radio, diet articles, and books—all are high-pressuring people to be thin, resulting in the frequent wail, "They're driving me out of my mind!"

That's basically the unwarranted, unhealthy alibi used by those who just don't want to cut down on calories or give up anything to achieve self-satisfaction. Hence they blame media pressure rather than admit, "I'd rather overeat than be trim." If that's how you feel, then accept the fact that you're overweight as your own decision, and live happily with it.

We don't put down anyone who is overweight—that's a personal choice, and we respect it. We don't aim to deride or bludgeon you. We don't assert psychologically or any other way that thinness guarantees happiness. But we do want to aid you if you need and want realistic help. The purpose of this book is to tell you, and anyone who is willing to follow the clear, simple directions, exactly how to slim down and stay trim—healthfully and Deliciously—no matter how many times you may have failed before. The *doing* is up to you.

If you blame media pressure as being one-sided in behalf of thinness, you're wrong. You'll realize that when you note that such pressure is small compared with the force of *billions* of dollars spent on food advertising and editorial matter in all media. That enormous, unflagging power focuses the spotlight primarily on rich, high-calorie food and recipes. The constant bombardment exhorts people to eat! eat! eat!—overshadowing any promotion of leanness.

Basically your *self-image* must govern your attitude and your actions. If you are overweight and like yourself that way, all good wishes to you—go well. If you don't like being overweight, now you have the sure, pleasant way to reduce rapidly and never be heavy again. It's your choice—you the individual, not "society."

You respond with justified resentment, "No, I'm not a 'people,' I'm a person." Right, we couldn't agree more. The purpose of our question, and your expected answer, is to impress on you the necessity of not allowing yourself to be governed by anyone who tells you that you can't do anything to help yourself over the long haul because most "people" stay overweight.

It's a fact, repeated endlessly, that you might as well give up on maintaining lifetime trimness because "most people, most women, most men, are overweight and stay that way." It's even more definite that *you* are not "most people" or "most women" or "most men." Their overweight problems aren't your concern. You are an individual, a person, not "most people."

Your weight control is your responsibility alone. The sooner you accept that psychologically, the sooner you'll make the decision to reduce and stay slim—or not. Other people can be whatever weight they want to be—that's fine with us. We co-authors, as individuals, prefer to be trim for a number of reasons: We believe we look better, to ourselves and to others. We know positively that we feel better. We are healthier and more active physically and mentally. We enjoy life more the slim-trim way. We stay lean by following through with Delicious Diet and Nutri-Slim Maintenance Guidelines. We, you, each of us, makes a personal decision.

Put the question another way: *Are you a statistic?* Of course not. So-called experts often quote research showing that anywhere up to 95 percent of those who take off excess weight put it back on again. Of course some people regain lost weight, but we've failed to track down reliable research on how many.

We have found that such figures are apparently "guesstimates," devised by people trying to sell a certain point of view. As Disraeli stated, "There are three kinds of lies—lies, damned lies, and statistics." Carlyle put it more kindly: "You may prove anything by figures."

The unfortunate psychological impact of these questionable "statistics"—that "X-percentages who take off weight put it back on again"—is that they permit many overweights to sigh with relief: "No use taking off weight because I'll only put it back on again." So they reach for extra helpings and the pounds pile on.

We know of a great many individuals (no percentages known or needed) who have reduced speedily with our methods and are still beautifully trim *years later*. Please put that in your psychological mind-set and be encouraged that you can and will reduce rapidly and never be heavy again: *You, the optimistic, thinking, doing individual*.

CAUTION: We must emphasize again, as we have elsewhere in this book, that if going on a reducing regime—whether D.D. or any other program—affects your emotional health deleteriously, *don't start the diet without seeking professional help*. Certainly emotional problems burden many people who are overweight, but reducing shouldn't be undertaken if you or your physician are concerned that it may cause mental illness or emotional disorders. Our firm advice in such a situation is to seek the counsel of a qualified psychologist or psychiatrist, and be guided accordingly. We urge that this treatment be on a personal, face-to-face basis with a specialist—who can give your problems the special attention they deserve.

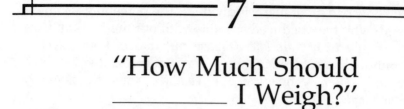

7

"How Much Should
_____ I Weigh?"

Our carefully reasoned answer to this question may shock you. From years of detailed research, study, consultation, and long experience in the field—analyzing "average," "desired," and "ideal" weights—our simple conclusion is this:

You should aim to attain and remain at the weight at which you personally decide you look best and feel healthiest, most vigorous, and lively.

The weight chart in this chapter gives the numbers that many medical authorities (not all) agree provide the best chance for good health for the average person. Guided by these numbers, providing a reasonable range, you select as your goal the weight you find is best for you as an individual.

It is desirable to ask your doctor for advice on what your ideal weight should be for your best personal health. If you are overweight, your physician has probably told you for years that you should reduce. For whatever reason, you just couldn't make it. Now you can, thanks to the *Delicious difference* offered by the Delicious Diet.

We urge you to follow this pleasant, taste-satisfying program to the letter for at least a week as a trial. When the numbers on the scale drop about a pound a day, that's your built-in willpower. You'll finally be on your way to achieving the trimmer figure, greater attractiveness, and better health you've long wanted.

WHY YOU ARE THE BEST JUDGE

As an intelligent adult, only you know at what weight you look and feel your best. You decide according to your appearance in the mirror, and your sense of vibrant health and well-being. If you deceive yourself by selecting as your goal a number at which you will continue to be obviously overweight and under par, then you fool no one but *yourself.* You're the one who will suffer most by not looking and feeling your best.

OVERWEIGHT IS HAZARDOUS TO YOUR HEALTH

It's not our purpose in this book to *scare* you into dieting and reducing lest you "drop dead," as too many self-seeking fanatics warn. You know that solid medical facts prove overwhelmingly that almost every individual has a far better chance for personal maximum good health and longer life if not considerably overweight. There's no guarantee, of course, but staying slim (not far underweight) is much healthier.

There is no question that a positive self-image contributes to good health. With the favored slim-trim appearance, you will enjoy the compliments of friends, as well as your own pleasing image in the mirror.

Because the Delicious Diet is well-balanced, it helps you to become most attractively slim, not unbecomingly gaunt. Its promise is pleasure, not punishment. You avoid even the slight risk of any loss of the desire to eat healthfully. As you lose weight rapidly you will be eating deliciously, without any sense of deprivation.

Every now and then, statements emerge from reputable sources bolstering the desires of some chubby people to believe that overweight is healthier. A recent *New York Times* story mentions a university scientist who said "the healthiest people are somewhat overweight." This was refuted in the same account in findings reported by Dr. William Castelli, director of the Framingham Heart Study, about the health of 5,200 Framingham, Massachusetts, residents since 1949.

Both studies showed that people who weigh the most (overweight) or the least (underweight) are most likely to die before their time. Both concluded that, when all factors are considered:

"Thin people live the longest." Repeatedly the facts are clear. The decision is yours alone.

PUT YOURSELF IN THIS PICTURE . . .

Starting right now, form this distinct picture to keep in your head as a constant reminder of the terrible health drain caused by carrying excess fat and flab. If, for example, you are 20 pounds overweight, picture youself filling a huge supermarket shopping bag with 20 pounds of large soda bottles, cans, and other heavy items.

Now, in your mind, carry that bulging bag with both hands supporting it at the bottom and walk out of the store. *Don't put down that 20-pound bag even for a second.* Stagger around with it, with no relief, whatever you are doing—at work, meals, talking with people, even sleeping under that heavy load all night long, then toting it around all day, day after day. . . .

Get the picture? Your back would feel as though it's breaking, your muscles aching, your lungs bursting due to the grinding effort. Think of how that crushing burden is ravaging your health

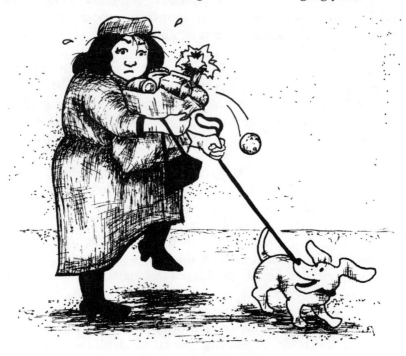

and well-being—not to mention draining away your looks. You may argue, "But I don't carry my 20 pounds in a shopping bag, it's distributed all over my body."

That's even worse, for the pounds of unrelenting fat are not only on but *in* your body—crowding your internal organs, putting extra demands on your heart and extra pressure on your spine, legs, your entire frame and system.

Whether you are 10 or 20 or more pounds overweight, keep in mind that picture of carting a 10-, 20-, or 30-pound shopping bag twenty-four hours a day. It will help you to start and continue dieting until you're rid of that awful, unattractive burden. Down to your desired weight, at last you'll be able to breathe more freely and be proud of your newly won health and good looks.

CHOOSE YOUR GOOD HEALTH, GOOD LOOKS, NUMBER

Now you're at the starting line, determined to slim down and stay trim for life—*for a better life.* You'll note that the following D.D. Weight Chart provides a range of numbers for your height— a desirable minimum and maximum. Those numbers are not fixed in concrete; a few pounds higher or lower are not significant for your best appearance and health.

We purposely don't list numbers for "small frame" . . . "medium frame" . . . "large frame." It has been our experience over the years that overweights overwhelmingly tend to designate themselves "large frame" in order to feel justified in weighing more than they should. Furthermore, there are too many individual variables to describe the type of frame accurately. A person could have "small" shoulders, "medium" pelvis, and "large" thighs and legs—defying correct categorizing.

Nobody knows better than you that if you fool yourself about your frame size and other measurements, no weight chart or reducing diet will work for you. Your happy bottom line, worth stressing repeatedly, is that *the Delicious Diet will work for you if you will work with it.* Just pick your right, winning desired weight according to the wide range listed. Stick with D.D., and you'll reach your goal deliciously.

Your own best number always is "desired" weight, not "average" weight. Because a dominating percentage of the adult population is overweight, "average" weight is not a reliable guide.

41

When the numbers are averaged arithmetically, the many over-weights overpower the relatively few underweights; the average obviously is far higher than desirable for maximum good health.

Another vital consideration is the amount of demanding effort a person expends at work, sports, and play hour after hour. Other factors too merit consideration. After all, we cannot live by numbers and statistics alone. A wise researcher commented that many statistical studies, especially on a large scale, have a way of "washing out most of the reality."

The Delicious Diet is created specifically—as no other diet before—to help you, the *individual*, slim down swiftly, healthfully, Deliciously—you, the individual, not a statistic. If you feel that at your age, or with your particular physical characteristics, you look better weighing a few pounds over the D.D. weight range for your height, or a few pounds under—then set that *personally* desired number as your goal. A few pounds more or less are not likely to affect your health adversely.

Now pick your personal goal number from this chart:

MEDICALLY APPROVED D.D. ADULT WEIGHT CHART
. . . DESIRABLE WEIGHT (COMPLETELY UNCLOTHED) . . .

WOMEN Range in Pounds	Height	MEN Range in Pounds
86–94	4' 8"	94–100
89–96	4' 9"	96–103
91–98	4'10"	97–105
94–102	4'11"	100–108
96–104	5'	102–112
98–107	5' 1"	105–118
100–110	5' 2"	110–124
106–117	5' 3"	115–130
111–122	5' 4"	120–135
114–125	5' 5"	125–140
118–130	5' 6"	130–145
120–135	5' 7"	135–150
126–140	5' 8"	140–155
130–145	5' 9"	145–160
135–148	5'10"	150–165
140–155	5'11"	155–170
145–160	6'	160–175
150–165	6' 1"	165–180
155–168	6' 2"	170–185

MEDICALLY APPROVED D.D. ADULT WEIGHT CHART
. . . DESIRABLE WEIGHT (COMPLETELY UNCLOTHED) . . .

WOMEN Range in Pounds	Height	MEN Range in Pounds
160–172	6' 3"	175–190
165–178	6' 4"	180–195
170–183	6' 5"	185–200
175–188	6' 6"	190–205
180–192	6' 7"	195–210
185–196	6' 8"	200–215

- *Weigh yourself every morning on arising,* giving the scale the responsibility for monitoring your weight. Unlike a well-meaning friend, your scale will tell you the truth, never lying to you. It's helpful to write down your weight each morning on the scale designs shown in Chapter 3 and elsewhere, or perhaps on a card in your bathroom. This will give you the encouragement of *seeing* up to a pound or more vanish day after day. (If you're traveling, or for any other reason can't get on a scale every morning, don't become frantic. Simply check your weight as often as convenient, maintaining your diet to the letter—and you can't help but lose pounds and inches delightfully.)
- *Weighing yourself unclothed* assures accuracy in the numbers each day. Otherwise, if you weigh yourself in Monday's clothing, then in heavier garments on Tuesday, the scale might vary three pounds or more for clothing alone. You certainly don't want to have to weigh your clothing separately.

A PERPETUAL PAYOFF

It's a glorious feeling when you get down to the weight where you look and feel your best, knowing that you have the way to stay trim at your most desirable weight from now on. Most of us go through stages of weight change; the wonderful difference for you through the Delicious Diet is that you' can be exactly where you want year after year. I know this from personal experience.

As a teenager, I was chubby and didn't like it, but didn't know how to trim down healthfully. Reaching my adult years, as a writer deeply involved with health and diet, I slimmed down and stabilized at 160 pounds. I met Dr. Stillman, tried the Quick Weight Loss Diet before co-authoring the book, reduced to 150 pounds, and maintained that. After he died at age eighty, I met Dr. Tarnower, slimmed down further on the Scarsdale Diet to 145 pounds, and stayed between 145 and 150 pounds.

On the Delicious Quick-Trim Diet, I dropped to 140 pounds, and enjoyed maximum vigor and alertness mentally and physically. That's where I remain with Delicious Nutri-Maintenance Eating. At times, during vacation and travel periods, I've gone up to 150 pounds, then go right back on the Delicious Diet. In a few days I'm down to 140 to 144 pounds again, feeling buoyant and energetic—the best weight for me, as affirmed by my doctor. I *know* that I'll never be heavy—I have the guidelines to keep myself trim, as you will have.

So . . . simply decide what is your personal best weight, then reach and maintain it Deliciously. You'll love the results. With the many inevitable problems in life, who needs excess fat and flab as an extra burden?

8

Before You Start
This Diet . . . Remember,
__You're Not the Doctor!

This is so important, it's vital that you read it now, up front, and follow wise counsel without question: It's a *must* that you check with your doctor before starting this or any other diet. We consider this point absolutely necessary—not just lip service.

If you haven't had a medical checkup during the past year, do it now. If you have been checked within the past 12 months and given a clean bill of health, simply phone your doctor and get approval to go on the Delicious Diet, giving basic details. You'll probably get immediate approval, since D.D. is such a sound way of reducing and eating.

You'll be doing yourself a good turn, dieting or not, when you have periodic medical checkups. In one instance, a friend told me that she was about to start one of my earlier diets. I asked, "Have you checked with your doctor?"

She replied, "I don't have to. Aside from being a little tired from dragging around this extra weight, and hating my overblown looks, I feel okay. I can judge how my health is. I haven't been to see a doctor for about three years. I'm my own best doctor."

I insisted. A week later she called and reported that the doctor's complete examination had led to further tests, which indicated a lesion beginning on one of her lungs. He told her that if she had waited another few months without care, medical treatment probably couldn't have arrested her lung cancer. "Maybe this saved my life," she said, adding brightly, "by the way, he said it's a great diet. . . ."

The Delicious Quick-Trim Diet is for adults in normal health.

It's not for growing youngsters, not for pregnant women, nor for individuals with medical problems. We couldn't be more serious about this—a medical checkup and your doctor's approval are essential before you begin any diet or exercise program. It can help detect and prevent serious, unrecognized problems from developing further.

Yes, a medical checkup may even save your life.

READ AND REAP THE MANY BENEFITS

Please read this book thoroughly, not just the daily diet details alone. Every word on every page is based on comprehensive and successful experience made available to you or anyone else for the first time. The clear purpose is to help you trim down most effectively, and to stay slim from now on.

Noting and absorbing every bit of information is the surest way for you to reap the greatest immediate and enduring benefits from the Delicious Quick-Trim Diet. Keep your copy of the book handy for repeated reference and use in the years ahead. Reading and rereading is vital for your healthier, happier future. You can look and feel your best always, with sustaining pride in your personal appearance and accomplishments.

On with your rewarding diet and fitness program. . . .

2

HOW YOU LOSE UP TO A POUND OR MORE A DAY —DELICIOUSLY

9

Detailed Delicious Diet
_____Guidelines
Don't Start Dieting Until
You Read Every Word Carefully

If you turn right to the diet chapters without reading, remembering, and then rereading these detailed guidelines, you'll be losing out on the maximum effectiveness of the Delicious Diet—instead of losing maximum overweight. Every word here and throughout the book is aimed to help you be your slim-trim best for life, not just temporarily.

Doctors have told us repeatedly, "Many patients simply don't follow our instructions, then blame us if they don't get well." Typically, a physician friend replayed a tape of an office visit in which he gave detailed directions to a patient. She murmured, "I guess I wasn't listening." Nor had she read printed instructions she'd taken with her. He said, "I can't help someone who won't help herself, can I?"

The same applies here. The Delicious Diet works for adults in normal health, no question about it. D.D. will work for you, but only if you follow these simple but vital guidelines.

D.D. GUIDELINES

1. Choose from the two diets—the Delicious Quick-Trim Basic Diet or the Delicious Quick-Trim Variety Diet. The fundamental difference between the two is that on the Basic Diet you may have chicken, fish, and the other foods on the daily listings, but _no meat._ This is important, since most meat brings along higher fat content. The Variety Diet provides meat, along with chicken and fish and the other foods listed daily, with a more liberal calorie allowance.

The choice is up to you personally, so long as you adhere to the guidelines. Both diets will reduce you swiftly and healthfully; the Basic Diet usually works a little faster.

2. *You may mix and match the two diets,* if you wish—choosing Monday on the Basic Diet, Tuesday on the Variety Diet, and so on, varying Basic days with Variety days, as you please, to fit your personal convenience. These diets are *personal* and *practical*, differing from any popular reducing diets offered before.

3. *Your dieting the delicious way is fully personal-choice:* You may follow the weekly listing for three meals of each day, Monday through Sunday, exactly as offered for each day—as most dieters do. Or . . . you may select any one of the seven breakfasts, any one of the seven lunches (or any one of the 14 lunches if you wish to include both the Basic and Variety Diets), and any one of the seven (or 14) dinners.

You may have Monday meals on Wednesday, or Thursday meals on Tuesday, as *you* wish. Since each day's meals add up to about the same number of calories (900 to 1,200), you trim down—whatever meals you select. Most Delicious Dieters prefer to follow the Monday-through-Sunday program in succession, just as printed. That's simple, satisfying, and effective in taking off excess pounds quickly. The choice is up to you.

4. *You have choices in the foods you eat.* If you are having fish for dinner, for instance, according to the listing you may choose to have it cooked any way you want (within D.D. guidelines) or prepared according to one of the Delicious fish recipes, which cut calories but not taste, so that you enjoy each mouthful thoroughly.

You don't have to use the Delicious recipes for each meal, although we think that you'll often prefer to do so. For example, if you have broiled steak in a restaurant, it's not likely to be cooked according to a D.D. recipe—but you can still remain within D.D. guidelines when you specify that you don't want it loaded with butter or rich sauce. Be sure to cut off all visible fat.

At home, if D.D. Onion-Stuffed Mushrooms are listed as a proposed dinner serving, you can substitute plain boiled onions; broiled mushrooms; stewed, broiled, or baked tomatoes; a cold sliced tomato, or whatever permitted vegetable you prefer.

The D.D. select-and-shuffle system enables you to satisfy your own particular taste each day, depending on whether you're in a mood for fish, or prefer chicken or any other D.D.-approved dish. *This eliminates the boredom factor that causes failure on most diets—but there's no danger of monotony with D.D.!*

Another Delicious individual-choice advantage is that you can benefit from the best food buys day by day. Where fruit is specified, you may prefer grapefruit when it is abundant and relatively low-priced, or strawberries in season, and so on.

Furthermore, you can save time and money by preparing an extra amount of food and freezing it for future use. With a Delicious muffin recipe, for instance, you might bake a dozen or more muffins and freeze the batch. Then you may remove one muffin at a time for your selected D.D. breakfast.

5. You don't have to count calories. By specifying permitted foods on the Delicious Diets and leaving out rich, high-calorie items, calories are automatically limited.

6. You don't have to weigh foods. Do limit yourself to *moderate* portions of the specified foods on your Delicious Diet. As an intelligent person, you know what a "moderate" portion is as opposed to a "large" or "giant" serving. If you eat oversize portions, you can't expect the diet to work, so you'd be deluding yourself. Keep in mind always that less is more—that the smaller the portion, the quicker you win better looks and a better chance for a healthier, more vigorous, longer life.

7. You may select and shuffle meals as you please: You may enjoy a Delicious "lunch" at the evening hour if you wish, or a Delicious "dinner" at noontime that day. Or you may have a "lunch" selection at midday, and another (or the same) "lunch" selection in the evening. But, obviously, you may *not* have two "dinners" (one at midday and one in the evening) on any one day—since "dinners" have more calories than "lunches." What could be less restrictive?

8. It's not necessary to eat every course listed: If you prefer to skip salad, vegetable, or fruit, or even a main course, that's fine. Nor should you feel compelled to finish every portion, to "clean the plate"; any calories left on the plate won't be added to your body. Learn to enjoy smaller portions, as in eating at a fine new-style French restaurant. Certainly the less you eat, the more quickly you'll lose weight—and so long as you feel well, it's fine for you.

The human body is a wonderful mechanism—if you're overweight and not eating enough calories to replace the calories you are using up hour after hour, *your body will pull the calories you need out of the fat stored in your body.* But, as noted earlier, if you keep stuffing into your body more calories than your system uses up, nature packs away those excess calories into "fat storage depots," causing your body to bulge.

9. *You may skip any meal if you wish* —preferably lunch or dinner, since breakfast calories are likely to be used up. Just be sure that you feel well and that, if you skip a meal, you drink plenty of water, or fruit juices, or other no-sugar-added liquids. The liquid is necessary to flush the "burned-up" wastes from your system. Many people have lived for weeks and even months without food, but not without liquids (or sleep).

No, we certainly don't recommend that you fast for days. But for the normally healthy person, skipping a meal is not likely to be harmful—quite the opposite. Just be sure you don't overcompensate afterward for the meal you skipped, putting back all the weight you took off.

10. *You may divide the daily food total into six meals a day,* if you prefer and find that convenient. It has been proved in many tests that an overweight person loses *more* pounds when consuming the same total of food in the day divided in six rather than in three meals or feedings. In this and every other way, Delicious Diets are adaptable to your needs.

11. *Eat only the permitted foods in each category,* as listed in D.D. daily menus. Those foods that are excluded are rich, high-calorie items (readily checked, if you wish, in the calorie tables in Chapter 18) as well as high-fat, salt-cured, salt-pickled, or smoked foods. Here are D.D. permitted foods:

FISH, SHELLFISH: All of the common fish and shellfish are relatively low-calorie and are permitted. When choosing higher-calorie fish—mackerel, pompano, shad, shad roe, etc.—eat relatively smaller portions. Always remove fatty skin and any visible fat before eating. In buying canned salmon and tuna, choose brands packed in water rather than oil (see labels), or wash off the oil thoroughly by placing the fish in a sieve and washing away most of the oil with running water.

Bake, broil, boil, or steam fish. Dry wines, lemon juice, and stock (bouillon, consommé, broth) may be used in cooking. "Fry" with vegetable cooking spray and no-stick utensils, not with fats. In cooking, fats (butter, margarine, oils, greases) are not to be used, except for very small amounts of sweet butter or vegetable oil occasionally (see Delicious recipes).

52

CHICKEN, TURKEY: Excellent, relatively low-calorie food: use as listed in daily menus. Always remove skin and visible fat before eating. Roast, bake, broil, boil, or steam. Don't use fats (butter, margarine, oils, greases) in preparation or serving, except for the slightest touch of butter or vegetable oil (see Delicious recipes). Duck and goose are higher in calories, and not permitted.

MEATS (on the Variety, but not the Basic Diet): Beef, lamb, veal, very lean ham and pork are permitted in moderate portions. Remove all visible fat before eating. Prepare and serve without fats (oil, margarine, butter, greases). Smoked meats in general are not permitted. Beef sweetbreads and brains are not permitted.

VEGETABLES: All are permitted, as listed on daily menus, including the wide variety of salad greens, except for these few strictly limited: Avocado, lima and kidney beans, canned corn, lentils, peas (unless a very small portion), soybeans, winter squash, sweet potatoes. A small potato is permitted on occasion, without butter. No fats may be added to any vegetables in preparation or serving, no fats (oils, heavy dressings) in salads. Low-calorie salad dressings may be used in very small quantities. D.D. dressings may be used, of course (see D.D. recipes).

FRUITS, FRUIT PRODUCTS: Fruits add variety, color, and texture to your meals, and are permitted where listed in daily menus, but *no* sugar added; no-calorie sweetening may be used, but it's better to ripen fruits, and enjoy their natural sweetness. No-sugar-added canned and frozen fruits are fine. Dried fruits may be eaten only in strictly limited amounts (they have a very high-caloric density). Fruits packed in sugar syrups are not permitted. No-sugar-added fruit juices are permitted in small servings. Watermelon is allowed in small servings only.

DAIRY PRODUCTS: *Skimmed* milk and nonfat dry milk are permitted in small quantities—a dash in coffee and tea, and very small amounts in cooking and serving. No other types of milk are permitted.
   Low-fat cottage cheese, low-fat pot cheese, low-fat ricotta cheese, and small quantities of farmer cheese (pressed cottage cheese) are permitted, as listed in daily menus. You may use regular creamed cottage cheese in smaller quantities if low-fat cottage cheese is not available.

Low-fat yogurt is permitted, but not yogurt with sugar added in the form of sugar-added fruit or sugared flavorings. You may use regular plain yogurt in smaller quantities if low-fat yogurt is not available.

Part-skim-milk cheeses are permitted only in very small quantities. The problem here is that "part skim milk" may be high in calories, since the ratio of skim milk to whole milk or cream does not have to be specified. A cheese may be high in calories although labeled "part skim milk."

Cream cheese and other cheeses made with whole milk and/ or cream are not permitted while on the Delicious Diet.

BREADS, CEREALS, GRAIN PRODUCTS: You may have a slice or two of bread a day (see daily menu listings)—small-size, thin-sliced bread or a small roll, also muffins (see D.D. recipes). It is preferable to choose whole-wheat or other whole-grain breads, protein bread, or gluten bread. Don't eat bread or rolls with a high content of sugar, honey, molasses, or rich-in-butter croissants while on the diet.

Whole-grain, low-calorie crackers or crispbread are permitted where listed in daily menus, only one, two, or a few, depending on size. Breadsticks, flatbreads, Melba toast, rye-toast wafers, and unsalted wafers are permitted. Crackers rich in shortening or other fats are not permitted.

Cereals, low-calorie, no-sugar-added dry and cooked types, are permitted as listed on daily menus. These include cooked whole wheat or oatmeal, 1 oz. servings or instant packets (100 calories or less). Dry cereals are permitted, but only types with 1 oz. servings under 100 calories (see calorie listing on packages) and with good bran content—such as bran, shredded wheat, Grape Nuts, unsugared puffed wheat. Serve with a little skim milk, no whole milk, no cream, no sugar added.

Rice, spaghetti, macaroni, noodles, and other pasta may be used as substitutes for potatoes where specified on daily menus. Plain rice and pasta are generally similar in calories to potatoes for comparable weights—and sometimes offer greater quantity. It's the rich, high-calorie additions such as a lot of butter, margarine, oil, cream sauces, and garnishes that make rice, pasta, and potatoes too high in calories for an effective reducing diet. You can enjoy them again in moderation when you're down to your desired weight.

SOUPS, BOUILLON, BROTH, CONSOMMÉ: Soups are permitted as listed in daily menus (see recipes too). D.D. Bouillon may be enjoyed at any time during the day. Limit your use of instant bouillon mixes (chicken, beef, vegetable, onion, etc.), even though they are under 12 calories per 8-oz. serving, if they are high in sodium (over 250 milligrams). Always read listings on packets. Low-sodium packets are available—or make your own—it's simple and delicious.

MISCELLANEOUS: Enjoy herbs and spices, and season your foods generously with lemon juice, but limit ketchup, mustard, pickle relish, and pickles. These may be low in calories but dense in salt unless you get "no-salt-added" brands (even then, use sparingly). If you use a little Worcestershire or soy sauce, or a few olives or pickle slices high in salt, be sure to omit other salt additives. If you add salt, or no-calorie sweeteners, use sparingly.

BEVERAGES: We recommend a glass of water with a wedge of lime or lemon, a refreshing and helpful drink, before each meal and between meals. Other D.D. "free" liquids may be substituted or added. Drink other liquids only as specified in daily menus. No-sugar-added juices such as orange juice and skim milk are healthful and nutritious, but add many calories if consumed throughout the day.

Coffee, tea: Drink as you wish in reasonable quantities daily, but no sugar added, and only a dash of skim milk if wanted; lemon juice in tea is okay. Decaffeinated coffee and tea are fine. No-calorie sweeteners are permitted instead of sugar, in reasonable amounts—but we recommend that you learn to enjoy unsweetened flavors. A wide variety of flavors in coffees (no-sugar-added) and herbal teas are available, and recommended in reasonable quantities. Real chocolate and cocoa drinks are not permitted, except as substitutes for a light meal, or in a very low-calorie version.

Sodas and flavored drinks: Drink no-salt seltzer rather than salt-bearing club soda, to cut salt intake. Artificially sweetened, no-sugar added carbonated and noncarbonated drinks are permitted, but only in reasonable quantities. No-caffeine beverages are preferable to colas and other drinks that contain caffeine (although not necessarily marked on labels); these no-caffeine beverages are now available, and are so marked on labels.

55

Alcoholic drinks: Dry alcoholic drinks are permitted in small quantities if wanted, but never sweet wines or sweet alcoholic drinks; see menu listings in following chapters. You may have a 3-oz. glass of *dry* white or red wine, including *dry* Champagne at lunch and dinner, if you wish. The nonalcoholic but refreshing D.D. Highball, made with mineral water, seltzer, or carbonated no-sugar soda and fresh lemon or lime, is permitted at any time.

Snacks: See menu listings in following chapters.

12. *If you are a vegetarian, you can adapt the Delicious Diets* to your eating requirements and needs very easily if you accept eggs, dairy products, and poultry; there are many other variations of vegetarians, as you know. Use D.D. menus and recipes, substituting vegetables and other items you permit yourself for other servings that you don't eat. You'll find D.D. vegetable recipes especially satisfying.

13. *Never stuff yourself.* No matter how little you think you may have eaten on the Delicious Diet (or any time), stop when you feel full. Overeating at any time can be a primary health danger. Overloading a truck at any one time can cause it to break down. Overstuffing yourself is a kind of self-destruction—*don't take any chances!*

14. *Don't take any "reducing drugs" on the Delicious Diet* (or on any other diet) unless prescribed by your physician—and then be sure to be checked by the doctor often).

15. *If you don't feel well at any time while dieting, stop and check with your doctor,* stating exactly what you've been eating. You'll probably be advised to go back on the diet after a day or two. If you don't feel well then, we strongly recommend a visit to your doctor. There is no logical reason why a normally healthy person shouldn't feel in top shape on a Delicious Diet, which provides a good balance of fine, nutritious foods.

16. *Regarding vitamins: Delicious Basic and Variety Diets are designed to provide sufficient vitamins for the average adult.* If you have special physical needs, however, you may benefit from taking a daily vitamin-mineral *supplement.*

17. *About fiber: The foods selected for the Delicious Diets are designed to provide natural bulk.* This increases your sense of satiety and aids digestion and elimination, particularly important to dieters.

18. *You should not feel hungry on Delicious Dieting.* If you do

think you feel a little hungry the first day or two, it's probably due to the change in your eating habits—those that led you to be overweight in the first place. Select from the lists of "feel free" choices to satisfy you until the next meal. The reaction might be psychological, too.

Just stick with D.D. After a few days, those feelings diminish and then vanish. Your appetite decreases naturally. Soon you won't feel at all hungry or deprived, and you'll savor the positive *enjoyment* of the Delicious servings you're eating—along with the surge of energy from dropping excess weight.

19. *Repeat Delicious Basic and Variety Diets week after week until you are down to your desired weight.* If you wish a change from dieting, switch to Nutri-Maintenance Eating for a week at a time, then go back on your choice of Delicious Diets. You may like to go on the Delicious Basic Diet one week, then the Delicious Variety Diet the next week. You may keep shuffling the two diets or diet days as you prefer.

20. *After you're down to your desired weight goal, don't continue dieting.* Your purpose is to get down to the weight at which you look and feel your best—and maintain that weight lifelong. Don't let yourself be underweight to any sizable degree, as that can be unhealthy. Losing weight is not a game. Read the detailed instructions later for maintaining your desired weight once you've lost the excess pounds.

If you start gaining weight again, go right back on your Delicious Diet at once—as soon as you see the Five-Pound D.D. Rerun Number on your scale in your morning weigh-in (details later).

21. *Read D.D. Guidelines as often as necessary, to make sure you are following detailed directions correctly.* If you deviate, you're not really on D.D., and you can't blame your diet for any failure in losing weight. The fact is that you are going to succeed in getting down to your desired weight deliciously and beautifully—like millions of others who have triumphed through this kind of nutritious, low-calorie way of shedding unwanted pounds and inches.

10

The Delicious Basic (No Meat) Quick-Trim Diet: Daily Menus and Recipes

Having read and absorbed the detailed guidelines in the preceding chapter (and also information in the earlier pages), you are ready to start Delicious Dieting and to enjoy delightful slimming in our, and now your, special way. You have a choice between the Basic Quick-Trim Diet (recipes in this chapter) and the Variety Quick-Trim Diet (recipes in this chapter and Chapter 11)—or you can mix and match from both, as you learned in reading the Delicious Diet Guidelines.

You can expect thrilling slimming results, as Sylvia Schur explains: "I have enjoyed the finest foods and wines in the world for the past thirty years as a food editor, and watched while friends who are top food writers grew rotund. Yet I never gained more than 10 unwanted pounds—*always taking them off the way now described in D.D.*

"Now, as people are being told by physicians to learn new patterns of diet, medically restricted to banish salts and fats, I continue to enjoy the D.D. way I prefer—the diet we now share with you. I appreciate this more fully right now, having shed 10 pounds to bring me down to my ideal—in just ten days of Delicious Diet cooking and tasting for you."

Delicious Diets are planned to help you enjoy life to its fullest—to meet each day with a sense of discovery and of appreciation for the promise it holds. When you wake up, spend some extra minutes on *you*. Before you dress for the day, go through some wake-up breathing and whatever physical activity you prefer (see Chapter 17). Enjoy your Delicious breakfast to start the day right. By following the rules exactly—*according to your D.D. personal*

58

choices—you are about to lose up to a pound or more a day. Go to it!

DELICIOUS BASIC DIET BRIEF GUIDELINES

1. *Simplest D.D. System:* Follow the week's menus for the three daily meals exactly, Monday's Breakfast, Lunch, Dinner, and so on—from the plentiful foods listed, no substitutes.

2. *Personal-Choice D.D. Method:* If you prefer, you can have any day's meals on any other day—Wednesday's meals on Monday, for example—mixing and matching meals as you personally wish.

You may choose any of the seven breakfasts on any day . . . any of the seven lunches . . . any of the seven dinners . . . on any one day.

You may have any "lunch" at noontime or in the evening, any "dinner" in the evening or at noontime, as you personally desire (fit the diet to your individual needs, rather than fitting your wishes to the diet)—but *not* two dinners per day. Yes, you may have two "lunches" (and no "dinner") on any day, if you prefer.

If you prefer to eat more *meat*, you may shift and shuffle the Basic and Variety Diets—Basic one day, Variety on another. You may mix and match meals from the two diets, giving yourself a personal choice between 14 "lunches" and 14 "dinners" from the daily listings of the two diets.

3. You may eat foods listed either using the D.D. recipes provided . . . or cooked any way you wish within D.D. rules.

4. Eat *moderate* portions of the foods listed, never "large" or "oversize" servings.

5. Don't eat all the food listed if you feel full or well satisfied—*stop*.

6. Skip any course if you don't feel like eating, but it's preferable not to skip any meal—especially breakfast. You might be likely to make up for meal skipping later on, with less self-control, and less efficient energy usage.

7. Drink lots of liquids, as much as you want in reasonable quantities: water . . . coffee, tea (preferably decaffeinated) . . . plain and no-sugar carbonated and noncarbonated beverages, any flavor (preferably no-caffeine) . . . bouillon under 12 calories per

59

cup (preferably low-sodium) . . . or all you want of home-made D.D. soup or broth (see Chapter 11).

A dash of skim milk in coffee or tea is permitted, also lemon and lime in tea and any other appropriate beverages. Don't substitute any beverages not listed.

You may have a 3-oz. glass of *dry* white or red wine (includes dry Champagne but no sweet wines) at lunch and at dinner, *if you wish*—preferably the lower-calorie dry "light" wines available. But you will lose weight faster if you don't have any alcoholic drinks. No other alcoholic drinks while on the diets; you may be able to drink again *in moderation* after you're down to your desired weight, as detailed in Nutri-Maintenance Lifelong Eating later.

8. Remove all fatty skin and visible fat from chicken, fish, meats, and other foods.

9. On salads, vegetables, and any foods, you may use D.D. recipes for dressings and other servings—but no high-calorie dressings, no regular mayonnaise, no extra oils, butter, margarine, or fats of any kind.

10. Keep dieting until you're down to your desired weight, repeating week after week—Basic Diet one week, Variety Diet the next week, and so on, if you prefer.

11. Weigh yourself each morning upon arising, and keep a record (see Daily Scale-Weight Chart, later in this chapter); if you're not losing up to a pound or more a day, you're not following the diet properly—check *detailed* D.D. Guidelines again (see preceding chapter).

12. Delicious Diets provide plenty of healthful, nutritious eating for the adult in normal health; if you don't feel well at any time, stop dieting and check with your doctor.

D.D. SHOPPING TIPS

These are for you if you eat at home, but even eating out, it's simple and enjoyable to follow the D.D. Guidelines—and to use these shopping tips whenever you do go to the stores.

- It's preferable that you try to arrange to visit the food market just once a week, with your menu plan in hand. Explore the new range of fruits and vegetables at the produce counter. Perhaps indulge in some varieties new to you, if available— especially low-calorie melons, kiwi fruit, and jícama (a potatolike vegetable popular in Mexico—it's extra crisp served raw in thin slices, for snacks or in salads, and only half the calories of potatoes).

- Also discover spaghetti squash, which looks like a yellow honeydew. After boiling, the flesh pulls out in strands like a heap of spaghetti—with about half the calories of pasta! Stock up on interesting salad makings, including a variety of lettuces, endive, watercress, radishes, jícama, Jerusalem artichokes (sold as "sunchokes"), alfalfa sprouts, sweet onions—all low in calories, delicious, and nutritious.

- Check both the fresh and frozen fish counter, and canned fish packed in brine. Buy your favorite breadsticks and wafers in whole-grain versions—preferably with sesame seeds—to make every calorie you buy and eat count for best nutrition and flavor. Check the labels of canned fruits you buy to be sure they are packed in water or natural juices, without added sugar. Check the frozen section for dry-packed berries with no sugar added, and for additional vegetable variety.

- Buy seltzer (it has no salt added), rather than club soda, which has higher sodium, and add no-calorie sodas if you want them. Discover a world of interesting teas with different flavors, and the variety in coffee roasts.

- Check your recipes and select the herbs and spices you will use to add deliciousness to your diet. Check the dairy section for low-fat and skim-milk cheeses—some of these will be low-salt as well . . . all to the good.

- You should find all or most of the foods indicated on the menus in supermarkets when they are in season. They offer interesting flavor accents that add little to your budget, particularly in comparison with high-priced, well-fatted meats, which you will avoid. If all are not available, choose D.D. approved substitutes.

- It's best not to buy foods prohibited on your diet—no snack cookies or candies, no red meats or sausages while you are on the Basic Diet, no ice cream or candy treats. Of course you'll make some exceptions for guests, children, and others, but none for yourself. You'll find that everyone will enjoy your wholesome D.D. diet snacks and meals—they're so delectable and don't taste like the usual dull, drab "diet foods."

Happy, healthful, *Delicious, and beautiful* weight loss to you. . . .

DELICIOUS QUICK-TRIM
BASIC DIET MENUS

BREAKFASTS

NOTE: Remember that at any meal you may substitute any comparable D.D. approved dish for a D.D. Recipe—for example, plain low-fat cottage cheese for *D.D. Herbed Low-Fat Cottage Cheese—and so on.

Monday

*D.D. Orange "Instant Breakfast" or Peach "Instant Breakfast" or chilled orange, cut into sections
*D.D. Herbed Low-Fat Cottage Cheese or *D.D. Caraway Cottage Cheese
*D.D. Molasses Bran Muffin or
*D.D. Whole-Wheat Bran English Muffin with *D.D. Refrigerator Fruit Spread or other low-sugar fruit spread
Coffee or tea

Tuesday

*D.D. Grapefruit Half with Cinnamon or plain chilled grapefruit half
*D.D. Huevo Ranchero or poached egg on 1 slice oatmeal bread, cut into triangles. (Where bread is specified at any time, it may be toasted if you prefer.)
Coffee or tea

Wednesday

*D.D. Nutmeg Baked Apple
Oatmeal or wheat cereal cooked with cinnamon stick, 5 raisins, 2 tablespoons low-fat cottage cheese or leftover brown rice heated with cinnamon and ½ cup skim milk
Coffee or tea

*See index for all recipes with asterisk.

Thursday

*D.D. Sliced Ripe Kiwi Fruit *or* 2 slices fresh ripe pineapple *or* canned pineapple packed in its unsweetened juice
*D.D. Skim-Milk Mozzarella cheese grilled on a slice of rye bread or whole-wheat bread *or* spread low-fat cottage cheese on bread or toast
Coffee *or* tea

Friday

Chilled orange cut in wedges
Cereal mix: Shredded wheat biscuit, bran cereal, puffed wheat, or any one of these alone, with sliced strawberries or diced apple wedge, and ½ cup skim milk or low-fat plain yogurt
*D.D. Whole-Wheat Bran English Muffin *or* a slice of whole-wheat bran bread *or* bread with a little *D.D. Refrigerator Fruit Spread
Coffee *or* tea

Saturday

Ripe mango sections *or* tangerine *or* other fruit in season
Whole-wheat or rye toast spread with *D.D. Herbed Low-Fat Cottage Cheese
Coffee *or* tea

Sunday Brunch

Fruit plate: strips of melon or pineapple slice; orange or grapefruit sections; berries; apple
*D.D. Egg Benedict Nouvelle *or* grilled herb cheese on 1 English muffin half
Remaining half muffin with low-calorie orange spread
Coffee *or* tea

Breakfast Alternate

In menu above, substitute poached egg on wheat-berry or whole-wheat toast instead of Egg Benedict Nouvelle and *D.D. Whole-Wheat Bran English Muffin.

DINNERS

We list dinners next, following breakfast, because that is a sound way to plan your meals. For most of us, it is usual to make dinner the best thought-out meal of the day—and it is often just as easy to make a little more for dinner, and to have the additional portion ready to use for lunch the next day. Or, if you are eating out, it helps in making lunch choices to plan what you'll have for dinner.

So here are your dinner menus, and you will find that not only do they flow from each other in preparation, but you will have some ingredient additions for breakfast, and some lunches ready to pack or to finish off in good style the next day. Of course, if you choose to have your dinner meal at midday, the lunch suggestions can easily serve as supper for the evening.

Monday

*D.D. Chicken Broth with Watercress *or* low-sodium instant chicken broth
*D.D. Chicken Espagnole *or* roast, broiled, or baked chicken with *D.D. Eggplant Zucchini Blend (Ratatouille) *or* *D.D. Herbed Spaghetti Squash *or* *D.D. Carrot Salad
*D.D. Simply Frozen Banana Pieces *or* *D.D. Frozen Green Grapes *or* sliced pineapple *or* kiwi fruit slices
*D.D. Mexican Coffee *or* tea

Tuesday

*D.D. Baked Flounder Florentine *or* Halibut Florentine
*D.D. Onion-stuffed Mushrooms *or* *D.D. Baked Nutmeg-Apple Summer Squash *or* fresh sliced tomatoes with basil
*D.D. Red and White Coleslaw *or* salad of your choice
*D.D. Lemon Whip
*D.D. Espresso *or* coffee *or* tea

Wednesday

*D.D. Herbed Vegetable Juice Cocktail *or* vegetable-tomato juice

*D.D. Gingered Stir-Fry Vegetables with Chicken or Turkey Strips
*D.D. Brown Rice Cooked in Broth
Chilled canned litchis *or* spiced peach *or* cantaloupe balls

Thursday

*D.D. Herb-grilled Trout *or* Whiting *or* other D.D. approved fish
*D.D. Bonanza Baked Potato, topped with a little yogurt, paprika, and chopped chives *or* *D.D. Spanish Rice *or* vegetable of your choice
*D.D. Caesar Salad Roma *or* Romaine lettuce and tomatoes *or* other salad with your choice of
*D.D. French or Italian Salad Dressing *or* other low-calorie dressing
*D.D. Pears Poached in Wine
*D.D. Orange Rind Espresso *or* coffee *or* tea

Friday

*D.D. Mixed Green Salad with sliced sweet onion and *D.D. Italian Salad Dressing
*D.D. Chicken Scallopine Diane *or* broiled chicken breast
*D.D. Broiled Tomato Half *or* scalloped tomatoes with basil
*D.D. Brown Rice Cooked in Broth
*D.D. Green Grapes with Crème Fraîche
Rosehip (or other) tea *or* coffee

Saturday

*D.D. Easy Clam Chowder with Vegetables *or* *D.D. Clam-Tomato Juice
*D.D. Scallops in Green Sauce *or* shrimp with spinach *or* *D.D. Shrimp Creole *or* other fish or shellfish
*D.D. Brown Rice cooked in broth with shredded scallion and cucumber, and tomato wedge garnish
Peach Halves with *D.D. Ricotta Crème *or* fruit compote *or* cantaloupe melon sorbet
*D.D. Espresso Coffee with Lemon Twist *or* coffee *or* tea

Sunday

*D.D. Asparagus Velvet Soup *or* low-calorie soup of your choice

*D.D. Turkey Breast Baked with Tarragon and White Wine *or* baked turkey *or* baked chicken
*D.D. Curried Rice with Lemoned Broccoli *or* other vegetable
*D.D. Nutmeg Baked Apple *or* *D.D. Real Fruited Gelatin
*D.D. Spiced Tea Punch *or* coffee *or* tea

LUNCHES

Each of these quick-to-prepare lunch menus includes some ingredients you are likely to have from the previous day or alternate pantry staples you probably have on hand. If you eat out, you shouldn't have any difficulty in getting these lunches in a restaurant. Enjoy!

Monday

*D.D. Curried Turkey Salad with Green Grapes and *D.D. Cucumber Salad with Crème Fraîche and Dill *or* fresh fruit salad and greens with *D.D. Orange Mayo *or* other low-calorie dressing
*Thin-sliced pumpernickel *or* whole-wheat breadsticks
*D.D. Spiced Tea Punch *or* hot or iced coffee *or* tea

Tuesday

*D.D. Lime-seasoned Chicken with Minted Carrot Garnish *or* cold chicken slices
*D.D. Eggplant Zucchini Salad *or* tossed green salad with *D.D. Italian Salad Dressing *or* other low-calorie dressing
Sesame breadsticks *or* whole-wheat melba toast *or* flatbread *or* Italian bread toast
*D.D. Lemon Iced Coffee *or* hot or iced coffee or tea *or* no-sugar soda

Wednesday

*D.D. Baked Flounder Florentine (cold) with grapefruit segment salad *or* *D.D. Vegetable Specialité with Zesty Broccoli, *D.D.

Baked Nutmeg-Apple Summer Squash, *D.D. Herbed Broiled Mushrooms, parsley-broiled tomato sprinkled with Parmesan cheese *or* choice of any three D.D.-approved vegetables
*D.D. Lemonade *or* hot or iced coffee or tea *or* no-sugar lemon soda

Thursday

*D.D. Stir-Fry and Rice Salad with Water Chestnuts and *D.D. Oriental Salad Dressing *or* *D.D. Seasoned canned smoked salmon *or* trout salad (with chopped carrots, celery, green onions, on bed of lettuce, with tomato chunks, zucchini spears, lemon wedges) and
*D.D. Creamy Cucumber Dressing *or* other low-calorie dressing
Sesame wheat crackers *or* whole-wheat flatbread *or* rice crackers
Hot Chinese tea *or* hot or iced coffee *or* no-sugar soda, any flavor of your choice

Friday

*D.D. Easy Clam Chowder with Vegetables *or* *D.D. Chicken Veg-etable Tomato Soup
*D.D. Sensation Spinach Salad *or* lettuce or mixed green salad
*D.D. Golden Dressing *or* other low-calorie dressing *or* D.D.-ap-proved mixed salad with lemon juice and herbs
*D.D. Molasses-Bran Muffin *or* slice of toast with *D.D. Refrigerator Fruit Spread
*D.D. Orange Spiced Tea *or* hot or iced coffee or tea *or* no-sugar soda

Saturday

*D.D. Herbed Vegetable Juice Cocktail with lime garnish *or* tomato juice *or* vegetable juice
*D.D. Chicken or Turkey Waldorf *or* sliced chicken or turkey with lettuce, tomato, radishes, cucumber slices
*D.D. Dill Dressing *or* other low-calorie dressing
*D.D. Minted Pineapple Chunks *or* other no-sugar-added pine-apple
*D.D. Cinnamon Iced Coffee *or* coffee *or* tea *or* no-sugar soda

If you have breakfast instead of brunch, add a light afternoon repast at under 200 calories. For example, *D.D. Spicy Seafood Salad with jícama slices or 2 kebabs of melon balls, pineapple wedges, and strawberries served with yogurt dip, and 2 *D.D. Sesame Wheat Wafers or "flatbread" wafers and *D.D. Ginger Tea Punch, *or* coffee or tea, *or* no-sugar soda.

DELICIOUS DIET SNACKS

The plentiful, satisfying meals on the Delicious Diets provide you with healthful nutrition as well as delicious taste. They should keep you full and feeling comfortable from meal to meal. Enjoy them slowly, savoring fresh flavors and contrasts in texture and taste. If you should feel a great need for nibbling on "a little something" between meals, we have listed some permitted low-calorie snacks and low-calorie foods for you in various chapters.

Keep in mind that even though the calories in these snacks are minimal, you must not eat more than *small* portions at any time. You'll lose weight more quickly if you don't snack—and, if you refrain from nibbling, you'll soon lose the habit and any feeling of need.

If you must snack, check the D.D. snack recipes particularly, or enjoy any D.D.-approved snacks of your personal choice. Beverages are a very good way of filling up, especially a cup of *D.D. Vegetable Broth or low-sodium instant broth in your choice of flavors (never more than 12 calories per packet, check labels). Note D.D. broth recipes in Chapter 11—you get some nutrients and a "full," satisfied feeling, *Deliciously*.

Other beverages include plenty of water (best for you) and, in reasonable quantities: coffee and tea (both preferably decaffeinated), no-salt club soda or seltzer, or no-sugar sodas in a wide choice of flavors.

Other snack possibilities are nibbles of raw vegetables, made delicious with D.D. dips, if wanted . . . cherry tomatoes . . . celery sticks . . . carrot sticks . . . green beans . . . zucchini strips . . . sweet-pepper strips . . . cauliflower buds . . . cold asparagus tips . . . fresh mushrooms and jícama.

Take advantage of the D.D. beverage recipes to help fill you up and satisfy any cravings between meals (your body should not be craving any extras, according to the experience of other Delicious dieters): Mocha Mint Coffee . . . Spiced Darjeeling Tea . . . Orange Rind Espresso . . . London Tea Punch, and others. Many herbal and spiced teas are readily available now in bulk or in tea bags, as well as flavored instant coffees—but, in both cases, check to make sure that there is no sugar content (if any sugar is added, they're not for you; you can always add your own no-calorie sweetening if wanted). With teas, a fresh lemon or lime wedge, or an orange slice, are always permissible.

You are now determined to get down to your desired weight. With the taste-satisfying composition and recipes of the Delicious Diets, you can succeed as never before when you follow the simple D.D. Guidelines faithfully.

However, if you slip off your diet for a meal or a day or more, *don't break down, don't scold yourself, and don't give up.* The trite phrase is true: Each of us is "only human." Guilt feelings, wailing about falling off a diet, are totally self-destructive. Instead, go right back on D.D. Based on the success of others like you, chances are that you'll then succeed wonderfully as you see the pounds on the scale drop day after day.

BRIEF TIP FROM A SUCCESSFUL D.D. DIETER

A beautifully slim and vibrant Delicious dieter said that she was inspired when she had a setback while dieting by the story of a small boy from a big city who moved to the country and was having difficulty learning to go barefoot. He complained, "I can't do it. My feet hurt. The rocks are too hard."

A country friend urged him to keep trying. When they met a few days later, the barefoot city boy grinned and remarked, *"Y'know, the rocks get softer every day."*

After a week on your Delicious Basic Diet, savoring the delectable tastes, oversized, oversalted, overdressed meals will seem to you just what they are—*overkill*. You'll be enjoying new eating pleasure . . . along with seeing your pounds and inches go down, down, down!

USE THIS SCALE-WEIGHT CHART

Weigh yourself first thing each morning upon arising (after relieving yourself, of course), before you dress. Write in your weight each day in the blank spaces provided on the Daily Scale-Weight Chart that follows here—for the first week.

If your weight isn't dropping about a pound or more a day (depending on how overweight you are), then you're not following D.D. Guidelines correctly. Review the listings again, and maintain your dieting *exactly* according to the detailed instructions.

Keep a day-by-day record while you're on the diet, and continue after you're down to your desired weight. Your scale is the best monitor—your daily weigh-in is your constant aid in staying trim and in looking and feeling your very best.

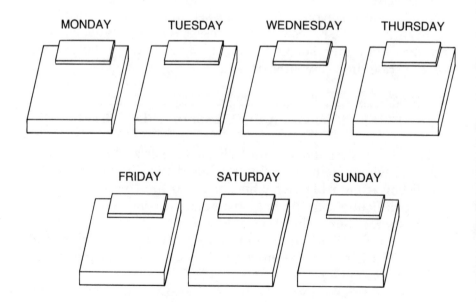

MONDAY   TUESDAY   WEDNESDAY   THURSDAY

FRIDAY   SATURDAY   SUNDAY

QUICK-TRIM MEAL PREPARATION TIPS

You will find all the meals for a week of the Delicious Quick-Trim Diet quick to prepare, as well as effective in shedding pounds. If you make some of the key recipes—vegetable broth, "mayo," or other salad dressings or sauces, these speed final preparations (complete directions are given in Chapter 12). If you prefer to buy already prepared sauces, broths, and dressing, that's okay, too. There are low-calorie and even salt-free versions of many such products now on the market.

When shopping, be aware, in making your choices, that packaged products called "low calorie" must now meet more stringent requirements for calorie reduction than those sold as "lite"—and choose accordingly. Be wary about unpackaged or loose "low-calorie" offerings that are not regulated and may actually be high in calories, sold by some specialty food stores or "gourmet shops."

Whether you buy convenience diet products or prepare your own, the recipes for a week of Quick-Trim menus are designed to provide seven days of satisfying meals that you will want to repeat often. They will help shape your new outlook and approach to food selection and meal preparation, while they help shape a new look for you!

D.D. FOOD PREPARATION BASIC GUIDELINES

In your food preparations for D.D., certain principles will be applied over and over again. These guidelines will always be valuable for you for good nutrition and delicious taste in *all* your food preparation. They apply to *all* meals and snacks, whether you are on D.D. or afterward—when you are trim—for family and company servings.

In the Delicious Diet system, you will enjoy good foods lower in fats and lower in high-cholesterol ingredients; very small amounts of oil and butter are used to carry flavors. We prefer to use sweet butter for the small amounts indicated—you will get richer flavor and less sodium. In some cases, certain oils are specified in very small amounts, for their special characteristics and flavors. For general purposes, we use polyunsaturated oil. In many cases, the remainder of what is normally oil or fat in a recipe becomes broth in the Delicious Diet approach.

WHAT ABOUT EGG YOLKS?

The egg is a remarkable package, from its perfectly designed shell (great for your garden compost) to its emulsifying yolk, and for D.D. its lean white. Since the white of the egg has 15 calories, and the yolk 60, we use mostly whites in the D.D. diet. To preserve extra yolks, freeze them in small waxed paper cups, each holding two yolks. These will make great mayonnaise, or Hollandaise sauce, or tender cookies or pie crusts—for non-dieters.

In recipes that traditionally use egg for binding or for aeration, we use a larger proportion of egg whites and less yolk. This applies to omelets and certain egg dishes, too. In place of egg for binding, a low-calorie cheese mixture may be used—we call this smooth blend of ricotta cheese and yogurt "D.D. Ricotta Crème"; in another version, cottage cheese is combined with yogurt or sour cream for "D.D. Cottage Crème." These basic recipes, as for most of those in D.D., are quick and make effective use of your double budget—time investment as well as dollars investment.

Because you will be eating less food, the nutrient density of each dish should be high, and you want good quality for the best flavors in the foods you choose. With our emphasis on fresh fruits and vegetables, whole grains, and on smaller portions of poultry and fish rather than more expensive meats, you may again find that you are saving dollars along with calories.

COOK'S TOOLS

While you can make any of these dishes without special equipment, a few good tools are well worth the investment. They also increase your joy in cooking.

A *food processor* or a *blender* are enormous assets in making these and other dishes quickly and with ease. You can also puree the cheese or vegetables through a food mill, or hand-beat mixtures for milk shakes, but you'll get faster and more effective results with the speed, sharpness, and emulsifying effect of the blades on a processor or blender.

A *microwave oven* is also an asset in Delicious Diet food preparation—although, again, not essential. Because it lets you cook and heat foods on serving plates, without added fat, the microwave oven simplifies and speeds both preparation and clean-up of many low-calorie dishes. One, or two or more, portions of vegetables can be prepared so that the essential nutrients are well retained.

Nonstick skillets also make it easier to prepare dishes with little or no added fat. One small skillet, about 6 inches, and one larger one, 10 to 12 inches, are recommended.

A *steamer*, a pot fitted with a perforated basket, enables you to cook foods in steaming vapor, without loss of flavor or nutrients in boiling water. This is especially effective for vegetables, fish, and certain poultry dishes.

A *pastry brush* is handy for spreading small amounts of oil or fat in a pan evenly, or to coat foods with oil or glaze for cooking. European cooks use goose-feather brushes, available at some specialty shops, but any small basting brush, or even a clean new light-bristled paintbrush, will do the job well.

Spatulas, rubber or wooden, are useful for stirring, folding, and pan-scraping.

Above all, two good, sharp *chef's knives*, one small and one large, are important for cutting and chopping. Learn to hold these correctly, the food cradled in one hand, with fingers curled under as a guard; the knife chopping or slicing with the other hand, as you "feed" the food forward. A *boning knife* with a slender, tapered blade is also important if you want to save money by boning chicken breasts or fish fillets yourself. And a sharp, serrated *bread knife* will enable you to enjoy thin-sliced hearty breads.

Until you are familiar with quantities of foods, use *measure spoons* and *cups*, even a *kitchen scale*, to ensure the accuracy of your recipes and the quantities you are eating. The number of servings given with each recipe indicates the correct portion size for weight loss. Savor the flavors of each dish, and avoid needless gobbling. *Delicioso!*

ABOUT FLAVORING

Herbs: You will enjoy the flavor of herbs in many of the D.D. recipes. To have these readily on hand, and for the pleasure of the process, it is fun and convenient to keep a pot of chives and perhaps little pots of basil, parsley, and mint—growing on your kitchen windowsill, to snip as needed. Fresh bunches of herbs keep well in a jar with a little water or in the refrigerator or as a bouquet on the kitchen table. Or use good-quality dried herbs, if you prefer.

Wine used as a flavoring in cooking is lower in calories than wine you drink, since the alcohol (naturally high in calories) evaporates in cooking, along with the calories.

Salt and sugar: We use little salt or sugar in these recipes. Flavors are balanced in the ingredients used, and sweet herbs or vegetables or fruits add sweetness. In some instances, a little honey is suggested. Since honey is sweeter than sugar, less goes further (all sugars contain essentially the same number of calories).

Serving: After you prepare your food, arrange it artistically on the plate. Plates with wide borders and a small well encourage you to enjoy modest portions, with full appreciation of flavor, texture, and the pleasures of eating.

Now, on to the Basic Delicious Diet breakfast, lunch, and dinner recipes . . .

BREAKFAST RECIPES

D.D. ORANGE "INSTANT" BREAKFAST

½ cup cold water or ice cubes
1 orange, peeled and cut up (or 3
   tablespoons frozen orange juice
   concentrate)

⅓ cup instant nonfat dry milk
   solids
2 tablespoons bran or Grape Nuts
½ teaspoon pure vanilla extract

Combine all ingredients in blender container, cover, and blend about 7 seconds, until frothy. *Makes 1 serving, 124 calories per serving.*

PEACH OR STRAWBERRY "INSTANT" BREAKFAST

In place of the orange, use 1 large ripe peach, peeled and cut up, or ½ cup hulled strawberries.

D.D. MOLASSES-BRAN MUFFINS

1½ cups whole-wheat flour
½ cup unprocessed bran
2 teaspoons baking powder
1 teaspoon baking soda
¼ teaspoon salt

1 cup buttermilk or low-fat plain
   yogurt
¼ cup molasses
¼ cup vegetable oil
2 tablespoons raisins

Combine flour, bran, baking powder, baking soda, and salt in large bowl. Combine in small bowl buttermilk or yogurt, molasses, and

(cont.)

oil. Stir into dry ingredients just until moistened. Add raisins. Spoon into oiled 2-inch muffin tins, until half filled. Bake at 375° F for 14 to 16 minutes, or until browned. Cool on rack. *Makes 18 muffins, 77 calories per muffin.*

D.D. OATMEAL WITH GRATED APPLE

Cook oatmeal as directed. Fold in ½ grated apple (skin on) and ½ teaspoon ground cinnamon. *Makes 1 serving, 159 calories.*

D.D. WHOLE-WHEAT BRAN ENGLISH MUFFINS

2 envelopes (or 2 scant tablespoons) active dry yeast
1½ cups very warm water (110° F)
1 tablespoon instant nonfat dry milk solids

4½ to 5 cups flour (half bread flour, half whole-wheat)
1 teaspoon salt
Unprocessed bran

Dissolve yeast in very warm water. Add milk solids, 2½ cups bread flour, and salt; beat batter well. Cover and let rise in a warm place for 1 hour.

Stir batter down; add 2 to 2½ cups whole-wheat flour, or enough to make a stiff dough. Knead on a floured board until smooth and elastic. Turn into a lightly oiled bowl, cover, and let rise until doubled—about 1 hour in a warm place, overnight in refrigerator. (If not ready to bake, punch down and refrigerate in a plastic bag.) Punch dough down, pat out ½ inch thick, and cut into 3-inch rounds. Dust both sides with bran, then let rise until doubled in size.

On a lightly greased griddle, over low heat, brown muffins on both sides. To serve, split with fork and toast. *Makes 14 muffins, 90 calories per muffin.*

D.D. REFRIGERATOR FRUIT SPREAD

1 ripe peach or 1 cup strawberries   Low-calorie granulated sweetener
   or 1 ripe pear   equal to 1–2 tablespoons sugar
Juice of ½ lemon or lime

Peel and pit peach or pear, or hull strawberries. Combine with
lemon juice and sugar substitute in blender or food processor container. Blend briefly, just until smashed. Serve or refrigerate in
covered jar, up to 3 days. *Ten calories for 2 tablespoons.*

D.D. NUTMEG BAKED APPLE

4 Rome Beauty apples   ¼ teaspoon freshly grated nutmeg
1 cup no-sugar ginger ale

Wash and core apples. Peel off a strip of skin just above the middle
of the apple. Arrange apples in a baking dish. Pour ginger ale over,
and sprinkle with grated nutmeg. Bake in a moderately hot oven
(350° F) about 25 to 35 minutes, basting occasionally with syrup in
pan. Cool. Serve with a little syrup spooned over each apple. (If
you own a microwave, 2 apples bake in 4 minutes.) *Makes 4 servings,
70 calories per serving.*

SLICED RIPE KIWI FRUIT

Kiwi fruit are fuzzy and brown-skinned on the outside, bright green
on the inside, with a tantalizing flavor reminiscent of a
combination of strawberries and pineapple. (If you haven't tried
them, they're worth seeking out.) They are ripe when the flesh
yields slightly to the touch. Serve simply cut in half, with a small

(cont.)

spoon. A whole kiwi has only 35 calories, and is a good source of vitamin C.

D.D. HUEVO RANCHERO

2 tablespoons water
2 tablespoons *D.D. Salsa or
  *D.D. Tomato Sauce
1 egg

Bring water and sauce to boil in small (7-inch) skillet, break egg into boiling liquid. Reduce heat to a simmer and cook egg 4 minutes, to desired doneness. (Or, to prepare in a microwave, place sauce in shallow bowl, drop egg in, pierce yolk with point of knife, cover with waxed paper, and microwave 45 seconds to 1 minute.) *Makes 1 serving, 85 calories per serving.*

D.D. EGG BENEDICT NOUVELLE

First, for the perfect poached egg: Bring water to a simmer in very small skillet (about 4 inches across). Crack shell and break egg into a small cup. Slip into simmering water. Reduce heat and cook 2 minutes. If desired, season with salt, paprika, or tarragon. Let stand 2 to 3 minutes longer, to desired doneness. Meanwhile toast English muffin half, place slice of tomato on this. Spoon finished egg from water and set on tomato. Top with *D.D. Hollandaise, or a sprinkling of grated low-fat cheese. *Makes 1 serving, 194 calories.*

D.D. HERB OMELET

1 egg
Salt
1 tablespoon water or buttermilk

1 tablespoon mixed chopped fresh
 parsley and chives
White pepper
½ teaspoon oil

Break egg and drop white into a wide, shallow soup bowl. Set yolk aside in half the shell. Add pinch of salt to the egg white and beat with a fork until foamy. Add yolk, water or buttermilk, herbs, and pepper, and beat all together with a fork. Heat oil in a 7-inch omelet pan. Pour the egg mixture into the hot pan. Shake the pan to distribute mixture evenly. Swirl with a fork, without touching bottom of pan, until no liquid runs to side. Let cook about 1 minute, until egg is set. Roll out onto serving plate. *Makes 1 serving, at 116 calories.*

POLYUNSATURATED HERB OMELET

Prepare omelet with ½ cup Egg Beaters egg substitute, add herbs as above, and ½ teaspoon oil. Cook. *Makes 1 serving, at 116 calories.*

D.D. BAGEL STRETCH

If a Sunday bagel is a treat with your omelet, cross-cut bagel into 4 thin slices with very sharp knife. Toast until crisp. Serve 2 thin slices per portion with *D.D. Herbed Low-Fat Cottage Cheese. *One bagel serves 2, 105 calories per serving.*

LUNCH AND DINNER RECIPES

Soups

D.D. CHICKEN-VEGETABLE TOMATO SOUP

2 cups *D.D. Chicken Broth or
   nonfat low-sodium chicken broth
¾ cup cooked vegetables, sliced or
   diced

1 cup tomato juice
2 tablespoons chopped fresh
   parsley

Combine chicken broth, vegetables, and tomato juice in saucepan.
Bring to boil. Sprinkle with parsley, return just to boil and serve.
Makes 4 servings, 60 calories per serving.

D.D. ONION SOUP BERMUDIANA

1 Bermuda onion, sliced thin
2 cups beef bouillon
1 teaspoon Worcestershire sauce

2 tablespoons low-fat Gruyère
   cheese, slivered

In a saucepan, cook onion slowly in 2 tablespoons of the bouillon
until tender and translucent. Add remaining bouillon and Worcestershire sauce; bring to boil and simmer a few minutes. Place
spoonful of cheese in each bowl, pour hot soup over, and serve.
Makes 2 servings, 83 calories per serving.

D.D. EASY CLAM CHOWDER WITH VEGETABLES

2½ cups *D.D. Vegetable Broth or
   canned vegetable tomato juice
1 medium onion, chopped
½ green pepper, diced
1 stalk celery, diced

1 can (10 ounces) minced clams
⅛ teaspoon dried thyme
Salt and freshly ground pepper
   (optional)

Pour vegetable broth into small saucepan. Add onion, green pepper, and celery. Bring to boil and cook a few minutes, until vegetables are tender. Add clams and thyme and return to boil. Taste and season with salt and pepper if indicated. *Makes 4 servings, 75 calories per serving.*

D.D. CURRIED TUNA BISQUE

¼ cup *D.D. Vegetable Broth or
   *D.D. Chicken Broth
1 scallion, sliced
1 stalk celery, diced
¼ medium ripe tomato, peeled and
   diced

1 slice apple, diced
1 to 2 teaspoons curry powder
1 can (3½ ounces) water-packed
   chunk-style tuna
1¼ cups low-fat milk
2 tablespoons *D.D. "Mayo"

Heat broth in small saucepan, add diced vegetables and fruit, and bring to boil, then simmer until reduced to a sauce. Stir in curry powder and cook a minute. Combine with remaining ingredients, in a blender or food processor container, and blend smooth (or simply stir together for a chunky soup). Heat gently, stirring, but do not boil. *Makes 2 servings, 152 calories per serving.*

D.D. MEDITERRANEAN FISH BOUILLON

1 cup *D.D. Fish Stock or clam
   juice
1 cup tomato juice
1 minced green onion, or onion
   salt to taste

1 clove garlic, mashed, or
   garlic powder to taste
Pinch each of pepper, thyme,
   paprika
Chopped fresh parsley

Combine in small saucepan fish stock, tomato juice, green onion, garlic, and seasonings. Heat to boil. Garnish with chopped parsley and serve. *Makes 2 servings, 45 calories per serving.*

D.D. GAZPACHO

1 cup *D.D. Chicken Broth or
   nonfat chicken broth
1 small red onion, peeled
1 green pepper, seeded
2 cloves garlic, peeled
1 cucumber, peeled and seeded

1 medium tomato, peeled and
   seeded
2 cups tomato juice
2 tablespoons lemon juice
Salt, pepper, Tabasco sauce

In blender or food processor container, combine broth, onion, pepper, garlic, and cucumber. Blend just until vegetables are chopped. Add tomato and whirl briefly until coarsely chopped. Pour into serving container. Stir in tomato juice, lemon juice, salt, pepper, and Tabasco sauce to taste. *Makes 6 servings, 35 calories per serving.*

D.D. MUSHROOM SOUP EPICURE

1 ½ cups mushrooms
3 cups *D.D. Chicken Broth or
   nonfat low-sodium chicken broth

½ cup *D.D. "Crème Fraîche"
Freshly grated nutmeg
Salt, white pepper

Cut stem ends from mushrooms and wipe mushrooms clean with a damp paper towel. Cut up and put into blender or food processor container with a small amount of the broth and puree. Add to remaining broth in soup pot. Add the "crème fraîche," heat, and simmer 3 to 4 minutes but do not boil. Season with grating of nutmeg and salt and pepper to taste. *Makes 6 servings, 47 calories per serving.*

D.D. CONSOMMÉ MADRILÈNE

After cooking and defatting chicken broth or making fish stock, boil the clear soup, uncovered, until reduced by half. This rich stock will jell naturally in the refrigerator. Or, if you prefer not to cook down, stir 1 envelope gelatin with one pint cold broth, add a tablespoon of tomato paste, then stir over moderate heat until gelatin is dissolved and mixture is clear. Chill and serve in soup cups, with lemon slice garnish. *Makes 2 servings, 38 calories per serving.*

D.D. QUICK CHINESE EGG DROP SOUP

2 cups *D.D. Chicken Broth or
   nonfat low-sodium chicken broth

1 teaspoon cornstarch
1 egg

Stir a little of the cold chicken broth with cornstarch. Add to remaining broth in 1-quart saucepan and bring to a boil, stirring

(cont.)

constantly. Reduce heat. Beat egg lightly. Pour in a thin stream into hot broth, stirring with fork. Cook 2 to 3 minutes, until fluffy strands form. *Makes 3 servings, 44 calories per serving.*

D.D. ASPARAGUS VELVET SOUP

1 can (1 pound) asparagus pieces
2 cups *D.D. Chicken Broth or
   nonfat low-sodium chicken broth

3 tablespoons *D.D. "Mayo" or
   low-calorie mayonnaise

Pour asparagus pieces with liquid into blender or food processor container. Blend smooth. Pour into saucepan, add broth, and bring to boil. Reduce heat and stir in "mayo"; heat through for a minute or two, but do not boil. *Makes 6 servings, 22 calories per serving.*

D.D. CHICKEN BROTH WITH WATERCRESS

½ bunch watercress
2 cups *D.D. Chicken Broth or
   nonfat low-sodium chicken broth

Grated Parmesan cheese

Wash watercress and trim off ends of stems; then cut leaves from the rest of the stems and reserve stems for other uses (chop into salads or cheese spread). Heat broth, add watercress leaves, and cook a minute. Serve with a sprinkling of Parmesan cheese. *Makes 2 servings, 30 calories per serving.*

Fish Dishes

D.D. BAKED RED SNAPPER FILLET CHINOISE

2 red snapper fillets (about 4 ounces each)
1 tablespoon soy sauce
2 tablespoons lemon juice

¼ cup *D.D. Vegetable Broth or nonfat low-sodium vegetable broth

Season red snapper fillets by dipping into mixture of soy sauce, lemon juice, and broth. Place in baking dish; reserve remaining sauce. Bake in moderately hot oven (400 degrees F) about 10 minutes, until golden, basting with remaining sauce and pan juice. *Makes 2 servings, 113 calories per serving.*

D.D. BAKED FLOUNDER FLORENTINE

12 ounces flounder fillets
Juice of ½ lemon
8 ounces fresh spinach
1 scallion, sliced
2 tablespoons *D.D. Ricotta or Cottage Crème

Salt, pepper, freshly grated nutmeg
¼ cup *D.D. Vegetable Broth or tomato juice
1 tomato, cut into wedges

Sprinkle flounder with lemon juice. Wash spinach, trim stems, and discard. Place in skillet with water that clings to leaves and sliced scallion. Cover and cook 1 minute. Place in food processor or bowl; chop with creme, salt, pepper, and nutmeg to taste.

Place 2 tablespoons of spinach mixture on narrow end of each flounder fillet. Roll up. Spread 1 tablespoon broth in bottom of casserole large enough to hold fillet rolls. Place rolls seam down in casserole. Garnish with tomato wedges, then sprinkle remaining broth over all. Bake at 350° F for 10 minutes. *Makes 4 servings, 196 calories per serving.*

HALIBUT FLORENTINE

Prepare as for flounder rolls, but place spinach mixture in bottom of casserole, top with halibut. Bake as for flounder.

HERB GRILLED TROUT OR WHITING

1 small trout or whiting per
   portion, cleaned
Ginger, fresh grated or powdered

1 onion slice
2 sprigs fresh parsley or dill
Teriyaki sauce

Season fish very lightly with ginger. Tuck onion slice and parsley or dill into cavity. Rub outside with teriyaki sauce and grill about 5 minutes each side. *Makes 1 serving, 150 calories per serving.*

D.D. POACHED FISH FILLET AND CARROT IN LETTUCE WRAP

1 pound fresh or frozen fish fillets
   (sole or flounder or ocean perch
   or other)
4 large romaine lettuce leaves
Salt, pepper, and dried tarragon
1 carrot, cut into slender strips
2 stalks celery, cut into slender
   strips

1 cup *D.D. Fish Broth or clam
   juice
¼ cup white wine
Bouquet garni of 2 sprigs parsley,
   sprig thyme, 1 bay leaf, leafy
   part of 1 celery stalk, tied
   together with twine
2 tablespoons *D.D. Ricotta or
   Cottage Crème

Poach the lettuce leaves in boiling, salted water 1 minute, until wilted and bright green. Remove and spread on paper towel to

(cont.)

drain. Divide fillets among leaves and season to taste with salt, pepper, and tarragon. Fold sides of each lettuce leaf in and turn ends up to enclose fish fillet completely. Arrange carrot and celery in bottom of a saucepan just large enough to hold fish fillets side by side. Add fish broth, wine, and bouquet garni. Heat to simmer. Set fish packages, seam down, on vegetables, cover pan, and poach gently 6 minutes, or until fish is just tender. Remove fish bundles to serving platter. Strain sauce and discard bouquet garni. Stir ricotta creme into sauce. Arrange carrot and celery strips around fish, then cover lightly with sauce. *Makes 4 servings, 158 calories per serving.*

D.D. SCALLOPS IN GREEN SAUCE

½ *pound spinach, or 1 package (10 ounces) frozen spinach*
1 *tablespoon *D.D. Fish Stock*
1 *onion, finely chopped*
¾-*inch piece of fresh ginger, peeled and cut into fine strips*

1 *green chili pepper, chopped (optional)*
¼ *teaspoon salt*
1 *teaspoon ground cumin or chili powder*
10 *ounces bay scallops or small shrimp*

Wash spinach and remove stems, then chop (or defrost frozen spinach partially and press out excess liquid). Set aside. Heat broth in saucepan; add onion, ginger, and chili and stir-cook until onions are limp. Add spinach and salt and cook until spinach wilts (about 2 minutes), stirring occasionally. Stir in ground cumin and scallops and cook, uncovered, for 3 to 4 minutes, until scallops are opaque and excess liquid evaporates. *Makes 3 servings, 120 calories per serving.*

D.D. QUICK SHRIMP CREOLE

¼ green pepper
2 cups *D.D. Tomato Sauce

1 package (12 ounces) frozen tiny
  peeled shrimp

Hold green pepper on fork over flame, or broil in hot toaster oven or under broiler, until skin chars. Remove from heat and pull off charred skin. Chop the peeled pepper and add to tomato sauce in 1½ quart saucepan. Add shrimp, bring to a simmer, and cook just until heated. *Makes 4 servings, 148 calories per serving.*

Poultry Dishes

D.D. GINGERED STIR-FRY VEGETABLES WITH CHICKEN OR TURKEY

½ cup *D.D. Vegetable Broth,
  divided
¾ cup thin strips of white-meat
  chicken or turkey
1 onion, sliced thin
1 cup thin-sliced mushrooms or
  celery
½ cup red or green pepper strips

½ cup thin-sliced carrots
1 cup green vegetable (broccoli
  florets, cut green beans, snow
  peas)
1 teaspoon chopped fresh ginger or
  ½ teaspoon powdered ginger (or
  more to taste)
2 tablespoons soy sauce

Heat 2 tablespoons broth in wok or nonstick skillet and stir-fry poultry 4 to 5 minutes, or until white. Add onion, mushrooms, pepper strips, and carrots and stir-fry in separate mounds in pan until glazed. Add remaining broth and green vegetable, bring to boil, and stir-cook all for 2 minutes. Add ginger and soy sauce. Cook, tossing to stir, another minute or 2 to heat through. *Makes 2 servings, 196 calories per serving.*

D.D. COQ AU VIN (CHICKEN IN RED WINE)

1 small chicken (about 2 pounds),
  cut up, skinned
Salt, pepper
2 teaspoons vegetable oil
4 small onions
1 clove garlic, minced
1 can (4 ounces) mushrooms

½ cup red wine
½ cup *D.D. Chicken Broth or
  nonfat low-sodium chicken broth
1 tablespoon tomato paste
pinch dried thyme
minced fresh parsley

Season chicken with salt and pepper to taste. Brown in hot oil in a heavy skillet. Add onions and garlic and stir over heat for a few minutes to glaze. Add mushrooms with their liquid, wine, broth, tomato paste, and thyme. Bring the sauce to a boil, then lower heat and simmer, covered, about 30 minutes, until chicken is tender, shaking pan and spooning sauce over chicken occasionally. Sprinkle with parsley. *Makes 4 servings, 222 calories per serving.*

D.D. CHICKEN CACCIATORE

1 pound boneless chicken breast
  meat, diced
¼ cup *D.D. Chicken Broth or
  nonfat low-sodium chicken broth
1 medium onion, diced
1 green pepper, diced
1 cup sliced mushrooms
½ cup minced fresh parsley
1 clove garlic, chopped

1 can (1 pound) Italian-style
  tomatoes with puree
2 tablespoons dry white wine
1 teaspoon dried rosemary,
  crushed
1 tablespoon chopped fresh basil or
  1 teaspoon dried basil, crushed
Salt, pepper

Cook chicken in nonstick skillet, stirring with fork until opaque and light golden. Add broth, onion, pepper, mushrooms, parsley, and garlic. Cover and "sweat," until onion is soft. Press tomatoes and juice through strainer and add. Add wine. Add rosemary and

(cont.)

89

basil. Cook, uncovered, over moderate-low heat about 10 minutes, stirring often, until blended and liquid is reduced. Adjust seasoning if needed. *Makes 4 servings, 225 calories per serving.*

D.D. CHICKEN ESPAGNOLE

1 chicken breast, split
1 cup *D.D. Tomato Sauce
1 tablespoon sherry

Pinch of dried thyme
4 spanish olives, sliced

Remove skin and any visible fat from chicken breast. Spread 2 tablespoons tomato sauce in small baking dish. Add chicken breast halves, sprinkle with sherry and thyme, and spread remaining tomato sauce over. Cover with foil and bake at 350° F for about 20 minutes. (Or cover with waxed paper and cook in microwave 6 minutes.) Uncover, garnish with sliced olives, and bake about 20 minutes longer in oven (2 minutes longer in microwave). *Makes 2 servings, 207 calories per serving.*

D.D. CHICKEN SCALOPPINE DIANE

½ pound boneless and skinless
*   chicken breast*
1 tablespoon flour
Salt, pepper, paprika

1 teaspoon oil
2 wedges lemon
2 tablespoons Worcestershire sauce
1 tablespoon chopped fresh parsley

Cut raw chicken in very thin slices, as for scaloppine. Dust chicken pieces lightly with flour seasoned with a little salt, pepper, and paprika. Heat oil in skillet and brown chicken slices quickly, just a minute or so on each side. Squeeze juice from lemon wedges over chicken pieces. Sprinkle with Worcestershire sauce and with parsley. *Makes 2 servings, 182 calories per serving.*

D.D. TURKEY BREAST BAKED WITH TARRAGON AND WHITE WINE

1 ½ pound turkey breast portion, (ready oven-roasted)
¼ cup *D.D. Chicken Broth or nonfat low-sodium chicken broth

¼ cup white wine
1 teaspoon dried tarragon

Place turkey breast in shallow roasting pan. Combine chicken broth and white wine and spoon half over. Bake 30 minutes. Sprinkle with tarragon and baste with remaining wine-broth mixture. Bake at 375° F 30 minutes more. Serve two-thirds roast hot for 4 portions; use remainder cold for salad or open-faced sandwich for two. *170 calories per serving.*

D.D. ROCK CORNISH HEN À L'ORANGE

1 Rock Cornish Hen (about 1 ¼ pounds)
½ onion, cut up
1 stalk celery, cut in pieces
Salt, pepper
2 tablespoons orange juice

2 tablespoons *D.D. Chicken Broth or nonfat low-sodium chicken broth
1 tablespoon chopped fresh parsley
Watercress for garnish

Stuff cavity of hen with onion and celery pieces. Season lightly with salt and pepper. Place on rack in roasting pan, then bake at 375° F about 15 minutes. Baste with orange juice combined with chicken broth. Bake another 30 minutes, basting once more with pan drippings, until golden brown and done. Sprinkle with parsley during last 10 minutes of baking. To serve, split hen in half, then place hen halves, cut side down, on bed of watercress. *Makes 2 servings, 256 calories per serving.*

To make 4 servings, use 2 hens and increase orange juice and chicken broth to 3 tablespoons each.

Vegetables

D.D. BROILED TOMATO HALF

2 medium tomatoes, halved
   horizontally

1 tablespoon *D.D. Italian
   Dressing
1 teaspoon dried basil

Arrange tomatoes in shallow baking pan. Brush with dressing, then sprinkle with basil. Broil 4 minutes. *Makes 4 servings, 18 calories per serving.*

D.D. ARTICHOKES VINAIGRETTE

4 artichokes
Juice of 1 lemon
1 clove garlic, peeled
1 tablespoon oil

4 peppercorns or ⅛ teaspoon red
   pepper flakes
¼ cup *D.D. Mayo
Red pepper strips

Choose compact globes, with fresh, dark green color. Wash artichokes between leaves thoroughly. Cut off stem ends with sharp knife; pull off and discard tough bottom leaves. Snip sharp points from leaves (easiest with a scissors). Place 4 artichokes upright in a deep saucepan just wide enough to hold them upright. Add lemon juice, oil, and peppercorns or red pepper flakes. Add boiling water to half cover artichokes. Cover tightly and boil about 30 minutes, until artichokes are tender (a leaf will pull out easily). Cool in broth. Spread top leaves apart and remove center leaves and choke. Stir mayo with ¼ cup of the artichoke cooking broth. Place 2 tablespoons mayo in center of each artichoke, garnish with a thin strip of red pepper. Dip leaves into center as you eat. *Makes 4 servings, 45 calories per serving.*

No fresh artichokes? Cook frozen artichoke hearts with a little lemon juice, clove of garlic, pinch of red pepper flakes, and spoonful of oil, plus water as directed on package. *Makes 4 appetizer servings.*

D.D. ONION-STUFFED MUSHROOMS

12 medium mushrooms
1 small onion, chopped

1 tablespoon Worcestershire sauce
1 tablespoon grated Parmesan
cheese

Cut off stem ends of mushrooms, wipe caps clean with moist paper towel, and twist out stems. Chop stems and combine with chopped onion, Worcestershire sauce, and Parmesan cheese. Pile chopped mixture back into mushroom caps. Place in small baking pan, or ovenproof dish. Bake at 425° F about 10 minutes, until mushrooms are browned and tender; or cook in microwave about 5 minutes. *Makes 4 servings, 28 calories each.*

D.D. EGGPLANT NACHOS MIXED GRILL

1 eggplant (about ¾ pound)
5 tablespoons *D.D. Vegetable
broth
2 tablespoons *D.D. Salsa
2 ounces low-fat mozzarella cheese

1 large tomato, halved
horizontally
2 tablespoons basil
4 mushrooms, washed and
stemmed
2 slices onion, chopped

Wash eggplant and cut off stem end, then cut unpeeled eggplant lengthwise into thin slices. Pour 1 tablespoon broth onto cookie sheet, dip each slice of eggplant in 2 tablespoons of the broth on both sides, and arrange at one side of cookie sheet. Broil one side 4 minutes, or until browned, then turn. Add to pan tomato halves sprinkled with basil and mushrooms filled with chopped onion. Sprinkle tomatoes and mushrooms with remaining 2 tablespoons vegetable broth and broil 4 minutes longer. Spread eggplant slices with salsa, then sprinkle with cheese. Broil all 2 minutes longer. *Makes 2 servings at 150 calories per serving.*

D.D. BROILED POTATO SLICES

Scrub potatoes (½ medium potato per person). Peel if desired. Cut into ¼-inch slices. Dip into cold chicken broth or water, then sprinkle with onion powder and paprika. Broil on rack on cookie sheet 3 inches from heat about 2½ minutes each side. *33 calories per serving.*

D.D. JULIENNE CARROTS AND CELERY

2 small carrots, peeled
2 celery stalks
½ cup *D.D. Vegetable Broth or
  *D.D. Chicken Broth

1 teaspoon *D.D. Herb Seasoning
  Mix

Cut celery and carrots into julienne strips about 2 to 3 inches long and 1/8 inch wide. In small pan, covered, cook carrots in broth for 5 minutes. Add julienne of celery. Cook carrots and celery, covered, for 5 minutes or until tender. Drain. Season with seasoning mix. *Makes 2 servings, 38 calories per serving.*

D.D. PUREE OF CARROT AND TURNIP

2 carrots
2 small turnips
1 small leek or scallion
1 teaspoon butter
½ cup *D.D. Chicken Broth or
  nonfat low-sodium chicken broth

Salt, white pepper, mace (or dash
  nutmeg)
2 tablespoons *D.D. "Crème
  Fraîche"
Fresh dill or parsley

Peel and dice carrots and turnips. Trim off roots and green portion of leek or scallion and wash thoroughly, peeling back top leaves.

(cont.)

Cut into slices. Heat butter in small saucepan and glaze vegetables, stirring often. Add broth, bring to boil, and season lightly with salt, pepper, and mace. Cook, covered, until vegetables are very soft, about 30 minutes. Puree in blender or food processor, or force through a sieve, adding enough cooking liquid to make a very thick puree. Beat in "Crème Fraîche" and mound in serving plate. Garnish with dill or parsley. *Makes 4 servings, 37 calories per serving.*

D.D. BAKED NUTMEG APPLE SUMMER SQUASH

1 pound yellow summer squash   *¼ teaspoon freshly grated nutmeg*
1 small tart apple
½ cup *D.D. Vegetable Broth or
   nonfat low-sodium chicken broth

Trim stems from summer squash and pare off any rough spots with vegetable parer. Slice squash thin. Core apple, then cut into very thin wedges. Combine squash, apple, broth, and nutmeg in small saucepan. Cover, bring to boil, and cook about 6 to 8 minutes, until squash is tender. *Makes 4 servings, 42 calories per serving.*

D.D. BROCCOLI WITH D.D. ORANGE MAYO

½ bunch broccoli (about 10   *2 tablespoons *D.D. Orange*
   ounces)   *Mayo*

Steam broccoli, covered, in a small amount of water until barely tender, 10 to 12 minutes. Drain. Spoon orange mayo over. *Makes 2 servings, 55 calories per serving.*

D.D. GREEN BEANS AND CELERY

½ pound green beans
2 stalks celery, sliced
½ cup *D.D. Chicken Broth or water

1 teaspoon *D.D. Herb Seasoning
Mix

Snip off the ends of beans. Cook, covered, in boiling broth, for 8 minutes. Add sliced celery and cook for 2 minutes, or until tender. Drain. Season with seasoning mix. *Makes 2 servings, 30 calories per serving.*

D.D. BROILED ONION

1 medium onion, quartered
  crosswise
1 tablespoon *D.D. Italian
  Dressing

1 tablespoon chopped fresh parsley

Place onion quarters in shallow baking pan. Brush with dressing. Sprinkle with chopped parsley. Place under broiler for 4 minutes. *Makes 2 servings, 24 calories per serving.*

D.D. VEGETABLE MÉLANGE IN FOIL

On square of heavy foil, layer thin slices of eggplant or zucchini, tomato, onion, green pepper. Sprinkle layers with broth or lemon juice, garlic salt, pepper, and basil. Close wrap with a double fold all around, grill or bake in very hot oven (425° F) about 15 minutes. *45 calories per serving.*

D.D. EGGPLANT-ZUCCHINI BLEND
(RATATOUILLE)

¼ cup or as needed, *D.D. Vegetable Broth or nonfat chicken broth
1 onion, coarsely chopped
1 clove garlic, pressed
1 eggplant (about 1 pound), cubed

1 zucchini (about ½ pound), sliced
1 green pepper, seeded and cut into thin strips
1 ripe medium tomato, quartered
1 teaspoon dried basil

Heat chicken broth in large skillet. Add onion and garlic and cook, tossing, until glazed. Add eggplant cubes and cook 5 minutes, adding a little more broth if necessary to moisten. Add zucchini and green pepper strips and cook 3 minutes longer. Add tomato, and basil, then stir and cook 2 minutes longer. Remove from heat and serve. *Makes 6 servings—4 for dinner, and enough for salad for 2— 38 calories per main dish serving.*

D.D. HERBED SPAGHETTI SQUASH

No spaghetti squash? Shred raw zucchini or yellow summer squash in the food processor or on coarse grater, and proceed as directed below.

1 pound spaghetti squash
2 tablespoons *D.D. Italian Dressing

2 tablespoons fresh chopped basil or 1 teaspoon dried basil or rosemary or herbs to taste

Pierce spaghetti squash with meat fork, to prevent cracking in cooking. Place in pot with boiling water to cover and cook about 25 minutes, until flesh is tender. Remove from heat and cool slightly. Cut in half lengthwise, remove seeds, and scoop out spaghetti-like strands with a fork into serving dish. Season with dressing and herbs. *Makes 4 servings, 22 calories per serving.*

D.D. STEAMED VEGETABLE PLATTER

Arrange in steamer basket, or on platter in microwave oven, *all cut to uniform size*: a center of broccoli florets, surrounded by mounds of green beans, carrot slices, yellow zucchini slices, or other vegetable of choice. Steam until just tender. Season with fresh lemon juice, fresh minced herbs, diced onion, and dash of cayenne pepper or paprika if you enjoy sweeter flavors. Top with a sprinkling (1 tablespoon per portion) of Parmesan cheese.

Side Dishes and Salads

D.D. SPANISH RICE

1 cup *D.D. Tomato Sauce or 1   ½ cup rice
   can (8 ounces) stewed tomatoes   1 bay leaf
½ teaspoon garlic powder   Salt and pepper to taste
¾ cup water

Combine tomato sauce, garlic powder, and water in a saucepan. Bring to boil, stirring occasionally to break up any large tomato pieces. Simmer 5 minutes, then stir in rice and bay leaf. Cover and simmer about 20 minutes, until rice is tender and liquid is absorbed. Taste and adjust seasoning. *Makes 4 servings, 128 calories per serving*.

D.D. BROWN RICE COOKED IN BROTH

Cook brown rice for time directed, using *D.D. Vegetable Broth or nonfat chicken broth in place of water. Add no butter or salt in the cooking.

D.D. RICE WITH ONION AND PEPPER STRIPS

¼ cup diced onion
¼ green pepper sliced into strips

2 tablespoons *D.D. Vegetable
   Broth or nonfat low-sodium
   vegetable broth
1 cup plain cooked rice

Sweat diced onion and pepper strips, covered, in vegetable broth until tender. Toss into rice and heat until warmed. *Makes 3 servings, 66 calories per serving.*

D.D. CURRIED RICE

1 cup rice
2 cups *D.D. Chicken Broth or
   nonfat low-sodium chicken broth

1 to 2 teaspoons curry powder
½ apple, diced
1 stalk celery, sliced thin

Combine rice in saucepan with chicken broth, curry powder, apple, and celery; stir well. Bring to boil and cook over low heat, covered, 20 to 25 minutes, until rice is tender. *Makes 6 servings (reserve 2 servings for Monday's salad lunch), 130 calories per serving.*

D.D. SPINACH LINGUINE WITH TOMATO-MUSHROOM SAUCE

¼ pound spinach linguine
1 can (2 ounces) mushrooms

½ cup *D.D. Tomato Sauce

Cook linguine according to package directions. Meanwhile, heat tomato sauce with mushrooms. Drain pasta and toss with hot sauce. *Makes 4 servings, 87 calories per serving.*

D.D. PASTA PRIMAVERA

¼ pound linguine, cooked
¼ pound spinach
1 clove garlic, peeled and chopped
1 small onion, peeled and chopped
2 tablespoons chopped fresh basil
    or 2 teaspoons dried
4 tablespoons *D.D. Ricotta or
    Cottage Crème

1 tablespoon grated Parmesan
    cheese
¼ pound green beans (fresh or
    frozen)
½ bunch broccoli, cut into florets
½ red bell pepper, cut in thin
    strips, or 1 tomato, cut into
    wedges

Boil linguine in lightly salted water, as directed. Wash and stem spinach leaves. Add onion and garlic, and cook 1 minute in water that clings to the leaves. Drain spinach well and chop; combine with basil, ricotta or cottage crème, and Parmesan. Steam beans and broccoli florets 2 to 3 minutes, until bright green and crisp. Drain pasta, toss immediately with chopped spinach mixture, cooked beans, and broccoli. Garnish with red pepper strips or tomato sections. *Makes 4 servings, 150 calories per serving.*

D.D. CARROT SALAD

1 large carrot
½ Golden Delicious apple, or
    other available eating apple
1 tablespoon chopped onion
2 tablespoons lemon juice

1 tablespoon *D.D. "Mayo" or
    low-calorie salad dressing
1 teaspoon chopped mint leaves
    (optional)

Grate carrot and unpeeled apple. Combine with remaining ingredients and chill. *Makes 2 servings, 54 calories per serving.*

D.D. HEALTH SALAD

Combine shredded lettuce, diced tomato, shredded cabbage (red or green), carrot slices, artichoke hearts, and alfalfa sprouts in bowl or container with cover. Before serving, toss with *D.D. French or Italian Dressing.

D.D. CAESAR SALAD ROMA

1 medium head romaine lettuce
1 slice French bread
1 clove garlic, mashed
1 tablespoon grated Parmesan
   cheese

2 tablespoons *D.D. Italian
   Dressing or low-calorie salad
   dressing
1 tablespoon *D.D. "Mayo" or
   low-calorie salad dressing

Wash romaine lettuce and crisp leaves in refrigerator. To prepare croutons, cut French bread into cubes. Spread in baking dish, cover with mashed garlic, and toast until golden. Arrange lettuce leaves on salad plate (the original Caesar salad was served with whole leaves, but cut them if you'd like). Sprinkle with croutons and Parmesan cheese. Combine Italian dressing and "mayo" and toss with greens and croutons. *Makes 4 servings, 23 calories per serving.*

D.D. MARINATED MUSHROOMS

Cut ends from stems of mushrooms and discard. Wipe caps with moist paper towel and slice. Toss with *D.D. Italian Dressing and chill in dressing to marinate.

D.D. RED AND WHITE COLESLAW

1 cup grated red cabbage
1 cup grated green cabbage
2 tablespoons grated onion
2 tablespoons *D.D. "Mayo" or
  low-calorie salad dressing

2 tablespoons plain low-fat yogurt
1 teaspoon caraway seeds
Salt and pepper to taste

Combine all ingredients, chill, and serve. *Makes 4 servings, 29 calories per serving.*

D.D. CHICKEN STRIPS WITH ORANGE SECTIONS

Use ½ cup chicken (cut into strips), ½ orange (in sections), and ¼ cup *D.D. "Mayo" per portion. Pile on lettuce, watercress, or celery. *209 calories per serving.*

D.D. CHICKEN SALAD WITH ALFALFA SPROUTS OR WATER CHESTNUTS

Use ½ cup chicken (cut into strips), ½ cup alfalfa sprouts, ½ tomato (diced), and ¼ cup *D.D. French Salad Dressing per portion. Serve on generous mound of lettuce and spinach leaves. *162 calories per serving.*

D.D. STIR-FRY AND RICE SALAD
WITH WATER CHESTNUTS

½ cup leftover stir-fry vegetables
½ cup cooked brown rice
2 water chestnuts, sliced, or
   1 stalk celery, sliced thin

1 tablespoon soy sauce
2 tablespoons apple juice or
   applesauce
Pinch of ground ginger

Combine vegetables, rice, and water chestnuts in bowl. For dressing, combine soy sauce, apple juice or applesauce and ginger. Toss with salad and serve. *Makes 1 serving (double the recipe for 2), at 144 calories.*

D.D. TUNA APPLE SALAD WITH GREENS

½ cup water-packed tuna, drained
1 tablespoon chopped onion
1 stalk celery, diced
½ small unpeeled Red Delicious
   apple, cored and diced

2 tablespoons *D.D. "Mayo"
1 tablespoon plain low-fat yogurt
1 tablespoon lemon juice
Lettuce, shredded carrot

Combine tuna, onion, celery, and apple in bowl. Stir "mayo," yogurt, and lemon juice to combine. Toss with tuna combination. Serve on lettuce with shredded carrot garnish. *Makes 1 serving, at 210 calories.* To prepare for 2, double all ingredients, except use 1 large unpeeled apple.

D.D. TUNA-MUSHROOM SALAD

Follow D.D. Tuna Apple Salad with Greens recipe, but use mushrooms in place of apple. If desired, season with a pinch of curry added to "mayo." *220 calories per serving.*

D.D. BOUILLABAISSE SALAD

Toss ½ cup canned shrimp with ¼ cup leftover *D.D. Red Snapper Fillet and its sauce, and small diced tomato. Serve on lettuce, with *D.D. No-Oil Dressing, 1 sliced olive. *174 calories per serving.*

D.D. STUFFED PITA BREAD

Cut 1 inch from top of small pita bread (reserve for making croutons or crumbs). Open out "pocket" in bread. Spread bread lightly with 1 tablespoon *D.D. "Mayo." Arrange 3 tablespoons shredded lettuce over bottom of bread. Add 3 tablespoons chopped cooked green beans, marinated in *D.D. French Salad Dressing and drained; add 1 ounce shredded feta or skim-milk mozzarella or other skim-milk cheese and 2 tablespoons chopped tomato. *198 calories per serving.*

D.D. RICE SALAD WITH STRIPS
OF MEAT OR CHICKEN

½ to ¾ cup boiled rice
¼ cup cooked meat or chicken
   strips
1 scallion, diced
2 cherry tomatoes, halved
3 green pepper strips

3 tablespoons *D.D. French Salad
   Dressing
Salt, pepper to taste
Shredded lettuce and spinach or
   cabbage

Combine all ingredients except greens in bowl. Toss to blend. Serve on bed of shredded lettuce and spinach or cabbage. *Makes 1 serving, at 200 calories.*

D.D. CURRIED TURKEY SALAD
WITH GREEN GRAPES

1 cup cooked turkey breast, cubed
¼ cup green grapes
1 cup *D.D. Curried Rice

2 tablespoons *D.D. Mayo or low-
   calorie salad dressing
2 tablespoons plain low-fat yogurt

Combine all ingredients, toss, and serve on lettuce leaves. *Makes 2 servings, 182 calories per serving.*

D.D. SALMON SLICES IN LIME JUICE

½-pound piece of raw salmon,
  boned
Juice of 1 large or 2 small limes
1 shallot, finely minced
⅛ teaspoon coarsely cracked white
  pepper

2 tablespoons fresh dill, chopped,
  or 2 teaspoons dried dill weed
⅛ teaspoon dry mustard
Watercress for garnish
Canned asparagus, seasoned with
  *D.D. French Salad Dressing,
  for garnish (optional)

Place salmon in freezer to chill for 15 minutes, until almost frozen. This will enable you to slice it paper thin, off the skin. Carefully spread salmon slices in a ceramic or glass dish. Sprinkle with lime juice, shallot, pepper, dill, and mustard. Cover with plastic wrap and set in refrigerator for 30 minutes or longer, turning and basting with juice occasionally. Arrange 3 or 4 slices on each serving plate, and moisten with marinade. Garnish with watercress and seasoned canned asparagus. *Makes 4 servings, 133 calories per serving.*

D.D. CUCUMBER SALAD WITH CRÈME FRAÎCHE AND DILL

1 medium cucumber
1 tablespoon white wine vinegar
  or rice wine vinegar
2 tablespoons *D.D. "Crème
  Fraîche"

1 tablespoon dill weed
Salt, freshly ground black pepper

Peel cucumber with vegetable parer; trim off and discard the ends. Cut into thin slices. Place in bowl; add vinegar, "crème fraîche," dill weed, salt, and pepper. Toss to mix. Chill 2 to 3 hours. *Makes 3 servings, 18 calories per serving.*

D.D. VEGETABLE SPECIALITÉ WITH ZESTY BROCCOLI

1 cup leftover steamed vegetables
¼ cup *D.D. French Salad
  Dressing
1 scallion, sliced

½ cup cooked broccoli
2 tablespoons *D.D. Zesty Tomato
  Dressing

Toss leftover vegetables with French dressing; sprinkle with sliced scallion. Garnish with broccoli topped with tomato dressing. *Makes 1 serving, at 93 calories.*

D.D. SENSATION SPINACH SALAD

2 cups washed young spinach
  leaves, stems removed, dried
  and chilled
1 cup sliced fresh mushrooms

4 radishes, sliced
½ cup *D.D. Golden Dressing
  (see below)

Combine all ingredients, toss, and serve. *Makes 2 servings, 51 calories per serving.*

D.D. GOLDEN DRESSING

2 tablespoons *D.D. "Mayo" or
  other low-calorie salad dressing
1 teaspoon Dijon mustard

1 tablespoon *D.D. French Salad
  Dressing or low-calorie French
  dressing

Combine and toss with salad or serve as accompaniment. *Makes about ¼ cup, at 43 calories.*

D.D. EGGPLANT-ZUCCHINI SALAD

Remaining *D.D. Eggplant-
Zucchini Blend from dinner

2 tablespoons *D.D. Italian Salad
Dressing

Stir ingredients together, chill, and serve. *Makes 2 servings, at 76 calories per serving.*

D.D. CHICKEN WALDORF SALAD

1 cup diced, cooked chicken meat
(fine use for chicken cooked to
make broth)
1 stalk celery, sliced
½ apple, cored and diced

2 walnut halves, broken up
2 tablespoons *D.D. "Mayo" or
other low-calorie salad dressing
2 tablespoons plain low-fat yogurt
⅛ teaspoon celery seed

Combine all ingredients, toss, and serve on lettuce leaves or watercress. *Makes 2 servings, 158 calories per serving.*

D.D. SPICY SEAFOOD SALAD

1 cup leftover cooked fish or
water-packed tuna, in chunks
1 stalk celery, diced
1 scallion, sliced

1 tablespoon *D.D. Salsa or
prepared salsa
2 tablespoons *D.D. "Mayo" or
other low-calorie salad dressing

Combine all ingredients and serve on lettuce, with a tomato and green pepper ring garnish. *Makes 2 servings, 150 calories per serving.*

Desserts

D.D. LEMON WHIP

1 envelope (1 tablespoon)
  unflavored gelatin
2 tablespoons (packed) brown
  sugar
Pinch salt
¼ cup cold water

¼ cup lemon juice
2 tablespoons nonfat dry milk
  solids
1½ cups ice cubes
Strawberries for garnish

Stir gelatin with sugar and salt. Sprinkle over water in small pan. Stir over moderate heat until gelatin dissolves and mixture is clear. Pour into blender or processor container. Add lemon juice, dry milk solids, and ice cubes. Blend about 6 seconds, until combined and light. Mixture will set very quickly as ice chills gelatin, so spoon immediately into serving dishes or champagne glasses. Garnish with a whole strawberry. *Makes 4 servings, 120 calories per serving.*

D.D. APRICOT WHIP

1 cup dried apricots, soaked
⅓ cup nonfat dry milk solids
Sugar substitute to equal 2
  tablespoons sugar

⅛ teaspoon almond extract or
  vanilla

To prepare apricots, pour boiling water over fruit to cover with an extra inch of boiling water at top. Cover, refrigerate, and let stand overnight. Drain, reserving ½ cup liquid. Place apricots and their liquid in blender or food processor container. Blend smooth, stopping and pushing apricots down from sides with spatula if necessary. Add dry milk solids, sweetener, and almond extract or

(cont.)

vanilla. Whip about 15 seconds, or until thick. Chill until serving time. *Makes 4 servings, 75 calories per serving.*

D.D. APPLE WHIP

Substitute 1¼ cups unsweetened applesauce for apricots and juice in recipe above. Add dry milk solids, sweetener, and vanilla, then whip and chill as directed. *Makes 4 servings, 49 calories per serving.*

D.D. ORANGE IN WHITE WINE

4 small navel oranges
¼ cup water
¼ cup white wine

Sugar substitute equal to ¼ cup sugar

Peel oranges with very sharp knife, discarding inner white pith. Reserve some of the outer peel, cut into slivers. Cut oranges into slices ½ inch thick. Reassemble, using picks to secure. Combine water, wine, and orange peel slivers in skillet. Bring to boil and cook a minute or 2. Cool and stir in sweetener until dissolved. Pour over fruit. Chill. *Makes 4 servings, 87 calories per serving.*

D.D. FROSTY SLICED ORANGES
IN SPIRAL JACKET

For each serving, peel a navel orange with spiral motion so that skin forms long loops (this is easiest to do with a sharp saw-tooth knife). Cut orange into sections, or slice, then replace in skin, winding into original shape. Place on tray in freezer about ½ hour to chill until frosty. Serve in the skin, to be peeled back as eaten. *71 calories per serving.*

D.D. INSTANT LEMON-BANANA WHIP

1 package low-calorie lemon
   gelatin or 1 envelope (1
   tablespoon) unflavored gelatin
   plus ¼ cup lemon juice and
   sugar substitute to equal ¼ cup
   sugar

½ cup boiling water
1½ cups crushed ice
1 small ripe banana, cut up

Put lemon gelatin (or unflavored gelatin plus lemon juice and sweetener) into blender or food processor container. Add boiling water, cover, and blend 5 seconds, until gelatin is dissolved. Add crushed ice and banana pieces. Blend 20 seconds, until smooth. Pour into individual dishes. Chill briefly. *Makes 4 servings, 37 calories per serving.*

D.D. BERRY WHIP

Use berry-flavored gelatin and 1 cup fresh or dry-frozen berries in place of lemon and banana in recipe above.

D.D. ORANGE MOUSSE

1 envelope (1 tablespoon)
   unflavored gelatin
1¾ cups orange juice
¼ cup orange liqueur
2 egg whites

2 tablespoons *D.D. "Crème
   Fraîche"
Strawberries, raspberries, or
   orange slices for garnish

Sprinkle gelatin over ¼ cup of the orange juice in small pan. Let stand a few minutes. Stir over low heat until gelatin dissolves. Add

(cont.)

remaining juice and stir to combine. Add orange liqueur. Chill the mixture until it thickens sufficiently to mound on a spoon, then beat until fluffy with a rotary beater. Beat egg whites until stiff and fold in. Fold in "crème fraîche." Spoon mousse into parfait glasses and chill until firm. *Makes 6 servings, 55 calories per serving.*

D.D. RASPBERRY OR STRAWBERRY MOUSSE

In place of the orange juice in recipe above, use ¼ cup water to dissolve gelatin and 1½ cups pureed raspberries or strawberries. Add berries to dissolved gelatin, then proceed with remainder of recipe as above. *Makes 6 servings, at 76 calories each.*

D.D. CANTALOUPE OR MANGO SLUSH

Peel ripe cantaloupe or mango. To each cup of fruit, add 1 table-spoon lemon juice and sugar substitute to equal 2 tablespoons sugar. Place in blender or food processor container and blend smooth. Freeze until like slush. If mixture freezes hard, break up and rebeat in blender or processor before serving. Serve ½ cup portions in Champagne goblets. *30 calories per serving.*

D.D. COFFEE GRANITÀ

4 teaspoons instant coffee powder
1 cup water
1 cup ice cubes
Sugar substitute equal to ¼ cup
*   sugar*

2 teaspoons vanilla
Orange rind twists for garnish

Combine all ingredients except for orange rind in blender or food processor container. Cover and blend 10 seconds until combined. Empty into bowl; cover with freezer wrap or foil. Freeze until firm at edges. Spoon into blender or processor; blend smooth. Freeze to consistency of slush. Serve garnished with orange rind twists. *Makes 4 servings, 6 calories per serving.*

D.D. MANDARIN ORANGE SHERBET

1 can (8 ounces) mandarin orange
  sections
2 tablespoons nonfat dry milk
  solids

Few drops almond extract or
* vanilla*

Turn mandarin oranges into bowl (with juice from can) and freeze until slushy. Remove to blender or food processor container, add dry milk and almond extract or vanilla, and blend until light and frothy. Return to freezer until slushy. Serve in goblets. *Makes 2 servings, 43 calories per serving.* For 4 servings, use 16-ounce can mandarin orange sections; double other proportions.

D.D. CHAMPAGNE SHERBET

2 cups Champagne
¼ cup sugar
¼ cup cold water
1 envelope (1 tablespoon)
  unflavored gelatin

Juice of ½ lemon or orange
Strawberries and/or kiwi fruit
* slices*

Set Champagne in the refrigerator to chill. Combine sugar with water and gelatin in small pan. Stir over low heat until gelatin is dissolved and mixture is clear. Stir in lemon or orange juice. Cool, then chill. Beat with rotary beater until foamy and light. Combine

(*cont.*)

in ice cream maker container with chilled Champagne, or combine in tall narrow container set in bed of ice and salt in larger bowl. Churn according to manufacturer's directions, or beat until frozen. If necessary to store in the freezer, beat again before serving. Garnish with strawberries and/or kiwi fruit slices. *Makes 6 servings, 64 calories per serving.*

IT'S THE BERRIES CHAMPAGNE

No time to fuss? Simply serve ¼ cup strawberries in a champagne goblet, or 1 ripe, peeled peach, topped with dry Champagne. What a way to celebrate vanishing pounds! *Makes 1 serving (your limit), at 95 calories.*

D.D. UNCOOKED APPLESAUCE

2 apples
Cold water
3 tablespoons lemon juice

Granulated sugar substitute to equal 2 tablespoons sugar

Core apples, then cut up and drop into bowl of water and lemon juice to prevent discoloration. In blender or food processor, blend apples with a few tablespoons cold water, the lemon juice, and sugar substitute until smooth. Serve at once. *Makes 2 servings, 95 calories per serving.*

D.D. GREEN GRAPES WITH "CRÈME FRAÎCHE"

⅔ cup green grapes
2 tablespoons *D.D. "Crème
   Fraîche"

1 teaspoon (packed) brown sugar
⅛ teaspoon ground cinnamon

Stem green grapes and arrange in 2 sherbet glasses or Champagne goblets, keeping tops flat. Spread each with 1 tablespoon "crème fraîche." Combine brown sugar and cinnamon and sprinkle over tops. Chill well before serving. *Makes 2 servings, 53 calories per serving.*

D.D. PEARS POACHED IN WINE

3 small Bosc pears (1 pound)
Juice of ½ lemon
1 cup water
½ cup dry red wine

3 whole cloves
1 piece cinnamon stick
1 tablespoon sugar

Peel and core pears, cutting into quarters and moistening with lemon juice to prevent discoloration. In a small, heavy saucepan, bring water, wine, cloves, piece of cinnamon stick, and sugar to boil. Add pear quarters and poach, covered, until just tender, about 8 minutes. Remove from heat and cool in the poaching liquid, then refrigerate. Serve 3 quarters of a pear per serving, with a little of the sauce spooned over (reserve any remaining sauce to flavor cold drinks). *Makes 4 servings, 96 calories per serving.*

D.D. REAL FRUITED GELATIN

1 envelope (1 tablespoon)
   unflavored gelatin
¼ cup water
1½ cups apple juice

¾ cup diced unpeeled red-skinned
   apple, grapes, sliced berries, or
   other fresh fruit

Off heat, sprinkle gelatin on cold water in very small pan, to soften. Add ½ cup of the apple juice and stir over low heat until gelatin is dissolved. Add remaining apple juice and cool until thick enough to mound slightly in spoon. Stir in fruit. Chill until firm. *Makes 4 servings, 58 calories per serving.*

D.D. OATMEAL CRISP COOKIES

1½ cups quick-cooking oats
¼ cup nonfat dry milk solids
2 tablespoons grated coconut
2 egg whites
Pinch salt

1 tablespoon lemon juice
2 teaspoons vanilla
4 tablespoons sugar
1 teaspoon grated orange rind

Combine oats with dry milk solids and coconut in large bowl. Beat egg whites until soft peaks form, then add salt, lemon juice, and vanilla and beat until stiff. Fold in sugar, 1 tablespoon at a time, and orange rind. Fold egg mixture into oats and milk solids. Drop by spoonfuls onto foil-lined cookie sheet. Spread gently with spatula into 2-inch circles. Bake in moderate oven (350° F), about 8 to 10 minutes, until golden. Turn off oven and leave cookies in oven to dry, about 10 minutes. Remove, cool on rack, and store in tin box. *Makes about 2 dozen, 39 calories per cookie.*

Beverages

D.D. LEMONADE

Juice of 1 lemon
1 pint water

2 packets granulated low-calorie
sweetener

Squeeze juice of lemon into small pitcher over ice. Sprinkle low-calorie sweetener over. Add water and stir to chill before serving. *Makes one serving at 29 calories.*

D.D. COFFEE

It pays to buy the best in coffee and enjoy natural great flavors, without the addition of cream or sugar. Even instant coffees come in a variety of roasts, including espresso—but avoid flavored and sugared pre-mixes. To enjoy the ultimate in coffee flavor, buy the best beans roasted to your taste, light or dark and rich; have them freshly ground, or invest in your own mill. Coffee beans store well in the freezer. Keep ground coffee in the refrigerator to preserve flavor. Brew coffee freshly, preferably in a filter pot without boiling, and if you want to enhance the flavor, add a dash of cinnamon, or twist of lemon rind. Some coffee beans and roasts are sweeter than others—experiment until you find your favorite.

D.D. TEA

Choose from a wealth of flavorful teas, brew with *boiling* water, and learn to enjoy the subtle difference in flavors without the

(cont.)

addition of dulling sugar or cream. In addition to tea varieties, from smoky Lapsang Souchang to sweet and light Jasmine or sweet, dark Earl Grey, explore the range of herb teas: gentle chamomile to tart lemon grass or fragrant rosehips, to satisfy your palate without caloric additions.

D.D. LEMON ICED COFFEE

Brew espresso coffee and pour over ice cubes to chill. Serve with lemon twist.

D.D. SPICED TEA PUNCH

Brew tea and steep with a twist of orange rind, 2 cloves, small piece of cinnamon stick.

D.D. MEXICAN COFFEE

Add a dash of cinnamon and cocoa to the coffee while brewing.

D.D. ESPRESSO COFFEE

Pour espresso coffee, brewed or instant, over an orange rind or lemon rind twist in each cup.

D.D. SLIM CAPPUCCINO

½ cup espresso coffee　　　　*Ground cinnamon*
½ cup boiling skim milk

Prepare very hot espresso coffee. Bring skim milk to a boil and pour the two together into a cup, quickly so that they foam. Sprinkle top with cinnamon. *Makes 1 serving, 46 calories per serving.*

D.D. COFFEE SLIM

1 cup cold water　　　　*⅓ cup instant nonfat dry milk*
1 teaspoon instant coffee　　　*solids*

Combine water, instant coffee, and milk in blender container or jar. Cover and blend or shake 3 seconds. Pour into a tall glass (over ice cubes, if desired). Sugar substitute may be added, if desired. *Calories per serving, about 85.*

D.D. CINNAMON COFFEE

Brew coffee, adding ⅛ teaspoon ground cinnamon to the pot, for 2 cups. Or place a piece of cinnamon stick in the pot while brewing.

D.D. UNCOFFEE AU LAIT

Brew coffee substitute (such as Postum) with steaming hot milk instead of water.

D.D. MIMOSA COCKTAIL

Fill Champagne tulip glass halfway with fresh orange juice. Top with low-cal lemon soda and a splash of Champagne. *Makes 1 serving, at 57 calories.*

D.D. CLAM-TOMATO JUICE

⅓ cup clam juice
⅓ cup tomato juice

Small lemon wedge
Dash of Worcestershire sauce

Combine juices. Add juice of lemon wedge and Worcestershire sauce. Serve over ice cubes. *Makes 1 serving, at 40 calories.*

D.D. HERBED VEGETABLE JUICE COCKTAIL

6 ounces *D.D. Vegetable Broth
  or vegetable tomato juice
½ teaspoon chopped fresh basil

¼ teaspoon chopped fresh thyme or
  dill

Combine juice and chopped herbs and stir vigorously. Serve chilled. *Makes 1 serving, at 36 calories.*

D.D. ALMOND SKIM MILK SHAKE

1 cup skim milk
2 tablespoons instant nonfat dry
  milk solids

1 tablespoon almond-flavored
  liqueur (Amaretto) or ¼
  teaspoon almond extract

Combine all ingredients in blender container or jar, cover, and blend until frothy, about 5 seconds. *Makes 1 serving, at 152 calories.*

D.D. BANANA OR PEACH SHAKE

1 cup plain low-fat yogurt
½ cup ice cubes
1 small banana or *fresh or water-*
  packed canned peach

Dash freshly grated nutmeg
1 packet granulated sugar
  substitute † (optional)

Combine all ingredients in blender container or jar, cover, and blend about 20 seconds, until smooth. Pour into extra-large glass. *Makes 1 hearty serving—2 cups (if desired, pour into a Thermos container to carry to work), 228 calories per serving.*

†A new sweetener, aspartame (called Equal), is not saccharin-based (and not cancer implicated). One packet equals the sweetness of 2 teaspoons of sugar, at 4 calories. It contains no sucrose, and is effective for cold drinks, particularly fruit- or acid-based—not for hot drinks or for use in cooking.

D.D. BANANA OR PEACH MILK SHAKE

Use 1 cup skim milk in place of yogurt in recipe above. *173 calories per serving.*

Appetizers and Snacks

D.D. CRUDITÉS WITH SALSA DIP

Carrots
Celery

Broccoli
*D.D. Salsa

Scrape carrots and cut into slender sticks. Chill in plastic bag in refrigerator. Wash and cut celery sticks, discarding strings. Chill in plastic bag. Cut broccoli florets, wash, and chill. Serve in attractive container, with salsa for dipping.

D.D. ZUCCHINI STICKS WITH HERB DIP

3 small zucchini
½ cup low-fat yogurt
½ cup low-fat cottage cheese
1 tablespoon chopped fresh chives

1 tablespoon chopped fresh parsley
1 tablespoon chopped fresh
* tarragon or 1 teaspoon dried*
½ teaspoon ground coriander

Scrub zucchini, trim off ends, and discard. Cut away any rough spots with vegetable parer. Cut lengthwise into wedges, then into 3-inch lengths. Chill. Place all remaining ingredients in blender or food processor container and whirl smooth, or mash and blend well. Empty cheese mixture into a bowl for dipping. Serve with chilled zucchini sticks. *Makes appetizer for 6, at 37 calories per serving.*

D.D. SIMPLY FROZEN BANANA PIECES, GREEN GRAPES, AND BLUEBERRIES

Ripe bananas, cut into 2-inch sections
Lemon juice

Green grapes
Blueberries

Insert a small dowel or plastic fork in each banana section to serve as handle. Quickly dip into lemon juice or ascorbic acid solution. Place on flat pan and pop into freezer. After freezing, wrap in plastic bags for storage in freezer.

Stem green grapes and blueberries and spread on cookie sheet to freeze, then tumble into plastic bags to store in freezer. *40 calories per serving.*

11

The Delicious Variety (Includes Meat) Quick-Trim Diet: Daily ___Menus and Recipes

Brief Guidelines for the Delicious Variety Diet are exactly the same as the "Delicious Basic Diet Brief Guidelines" at the beginning of Chapter 10. Please read those guidelines carefully and follow them exactly in enjoying the Daily Menus for the Variety Diet that follows.

DELICIOUS QUICK-TRIM VARIETY DIET

BREAKFASTS

Eat according to the Delicious Quick-Trim Basic breakfasts in Chapter 10. The breakfast menus are created to be tasty, satisfying, and effective for both the Basic and Variety diets.

DINNERS

NOTE: As always on Delicious Diets, you may substitute your own choice of dishes for any D.D. recipes (whether eating at home or out)—as long as you stay within D.D. Guidelines. For example, instead of D.D. Veal or Turkey Scaloppine alla Marsala, you may have any veal or turkey dish, such as Roast Turkey, but always remove skin and any visible fat from poultry and meats. Of course, if you're eating out, always order *without* heavy gravies, sauces, and dressings.

Monday

*D.D. Zucchini Sticks with Herb Dip
*D.D. Veal or Turkey Scaloppine alla Marsala *or* *D.D. Lean Beef or Veal Burger *or* D.D.-approved beef, veal, or turkey dish
*D.D. Julienne of Carrots and Celery
*D.D. Spinach Linguine or other pasta or rice with Tomato Mushroom Sauce *or* other D.D.-approved vegetables
*D.D. Coffee Granità *or* D.D.-approved fruit
*D.D. Slim Cappuccino *or* other coffee or tea

Tuesday

*D.D. Clam-Tomato Juice
*D.D. Baked Red Snapper Fillet Chinoise *or* your choice of other fish fillet
*D.D. Rice with Onion and Pepper Strips *or* Chinese Vegetables with Ginger
*D.D. Mandarin Orange Sherbet *or* chilled mandarin orange or tangerine sections
Lemon grass tea *or* other tea or *D.D. Lemonade

Wednesday

*D.D. Onion Soup Bermudiana (1 cup) *or* low-sodium instant onion broth *or* other broth of your choice
*D.D. Lamb or Veal Kebabs with Onions, Pepper Squares, and Mushrooms *or* *D.D. Chops Italienne, fat trimmed
*D.D. Broiled Potato Slices *or* broiled new potato with chives
*D.D. Broiled Tomato Half *or* broiled zucchini sticks
*D.D. Apricot Whip *or* *D.D. Apple Whip *or* crisp fresh apple with honey yogurt dip
*D.D. Cinnamon Coffee *or* coffee or tea

Thursday

*D.D. Chicken Cacciatore *or* other D.D.-approved veal or chicken
*D.D. Herbed Spaghetti Squash *or* boiled rice
Shredded lettuce and cucumber with *D.D. Italian Salad Dressing
*D.D. Orange in White Wine *or* *D.D. Frosty Sliced Orange in Spiral
   Jacket
*D.D. Espresso Coffee *or* *D.D. Slim Cappuccino *or* iced tea

Friday

*D.D. Mediterranean Fish Bouillon *or* *D.D. Gazpacho *or* *D.D.
   Vegetable Broth
*D.D. Poached Fish Fillet and Carrot in Lettuce Wrap *or* the same
   dish made with flounder fillets *or* pan-poached trout or other
   D.D.-approved fish
*D.D. Sensation Spinach Salad *or* *D.D. Garden Veggie Slaw
*D.D. Instant Lemon-Banana Whip *or* Lemon Bavarian *or* *D.D.
   Berry Whip
Almond coffee *or* coffee or tea of choice

Saturday

*D.D. Mushroom Soup Epicure *or* low-sodium broth with sliced
   mushrooms
*D.D. London Broil *or* *D.D. Green Pepper Steak *or* other D.D.-
   approved meat
*D.D. Broccoli with *D.D. Orange Mayo *or* *D.D. Broiled Onions
Cherry Tomato Watercress Salad with *D.D. Green Goddess Dress-
   ing or other low-calorie dressing
*D.D. Orange Mousse *or* *D.D. Raspberry or Strawberry Mousse
*D.D. Cinnamon Coffee *or* coffee or minted tea

Sunday

*D.D. Artichoke Vinaigrette
*D.D. Coq au Vin *or* *D.D. Rock Cornish Hen à l'Orange *or* other
   D.D.-approved chicken or turkey
*D.D. Puree of Carrot and Turnip

*D.D. Green Beans and Celery *or* green salad with shredded beets and walnuts and *D.D. French Dressing
*D.D. Yogurt Cheese Pie *or* fruited *D.D. Ricotta Crème
Demi-tasse *or* coffee or tea, regular or herb

LUNCHES

Monday

*D.D. Gazpacho *or* *D.D. Consommé Madrilène
*D.D. Chicken Strips and Orange Sections, with Boston lettuce, watercress, or celery, marinated green beans, and *D.D. "Mayo" *or* *D.D. Chicken Salad with alfalfa sprouts (and/or bean sprouts) or water chestnuts *or* other D.D.-approved cold chicken
Rye wafer or sesame cracker
Ripe pear or crisp apple *or* other D.D.-approved fruit
Coffee *or* tea

Tuesday

*D.D. Rice Salad with Strips of Meat or Chicken (from dinner), with cherry tomatoes, peppers, and *D.D. Vinaigrette Dressing *or* other D.D.-approved salad
Sesame Melba toast or breadsticks or flatbread
Melon wedge with lemon
*D.D. Coffee Slim (iced) *or* coffee or tea of choice

Wednesday

*D.D. Quick Chinese Egg Drop Soup
*D.D. Tuna-Fruit Salad with Greens *or* *D.D. Tuna Mushroom Salad *or* sardines packed in mustard sauce with romaine lettuce, sliced tomato, and marinated green beans
*D.D. Oatmeal Crisp Cookie
*D.D. Spiced Tea Punch *or* hot or iced coffee or tea *or* no-sugar soda

Thursday

*D.D. Stuffed Pita Bread (with shredded lettuce, chopped tomatoes, marinated green beans, any other vegetables on hand, topped with crumbled feta or Swiss cheese and *D.D. "Mayo" *or* other D.D.-approved vegetables with pita bread or slice of whole-wheat toast

Carrot sticks, celery sticks, jícama sticks

Plain low-fat yogurt with *D.D. Refrigerator Fruit Spread *or* coffee yogurt

Friday

*D.D. Bouillabaisse Salad *or* other D.D.-approved salad

Frozen pineapple slices *or* *D.D. Simply Frozen Green Grapes *or* minted canned pineapple

D.D. Spiced Tea *or* hot or iced coffee or tea *or* no-calorie soda

Saturday

*D.D. Salmon Slices in Lime Juice *or* tuna with asparagus vinaigrette *or* D.D. Dinner-Bonus Fish *or* other D.D.-approved salmon or tuna salad

Sesame whole-wheat cracker *or* slice of whole-wheat toast

*D.D. Cantaloupe Slush *or* *D.D. Mango Slush *or* *D.D. Simply Frozen Banana Pieces

Sunday Brunch

*D.D. Mimosa Cocktail *or* D.D.-approved juice

*D.D. Herb Omelet *or* Mushroom Omelet *or* Spanish Omelet

*D.D. Bagel Stretch with Neufchâtel cheese *or* No-Sugar Peach-Lime Spread *or* low-fat cottage cheese

Coffee *or* tea

POULTRY AND MEAT DISHES

These accentuate the light—in calories and in cost. For example, make Scaloppine alla Marsala as a main dish, using choice veal, or with equally tender but far less expensive white turkey meat cut into thin slices.

VEAL OR TURKEY SCALOPPINE ALLA MARSALA

¾ pound thin-sliced lean veal or
    turkey breast
1 tablespoon flour
Salt, pepper, paprika

2 teaspoons vegetable oil
⅓ cup Marsala wine
1 can (6 ounces) mushrooms
Lemon Wedges for garnish

Dust scaloppine with flour combined with seasonings. Pound with a mallet or the edge of a plate to flatten. Heat oil in nonstick skillet and brown meat slices on both sides. Add Marsala and mushrooms with liquid and simmer uncovered until tender, about 15 minutes. Serve with sauce spooned over, and a lemon wedge garnish. *Makes 4 servings, 210 calories per serving.*

D.D. LEAN BEEF OR VEAL BURGER

½ pound ground lean beef or veal
    shoulder
2 tablespoons water
2 tablespoons minced onion

Salt, pepper, ground cloves
2 tablespoons Dijon mustard
1 tablespoon *D.D. No-Oil
    Dressing or *D.D. "Mayo"

Combine meat with water, onion, salt, pepper, and a pinch of cloves. Form into 2 hamburger patties. Cook in hot nonstick pan

(cont.)

5 minutes each side for medium rare. Combine mustard and salad dressing and spread on burgers. *Makes 2 servings, 228 calories per serving.*

D.D. LAMB OR VEAL KEBABS WITH ONIONS, PEPPER SQUARES, AND MUSHROOMS

¾ pound lean boneless lamb or veal leg
¼ cup wine vinegar
1 tablespoon oil
*¼ cup *D.D. Chicken Broth or nonfat low-sodium chicken broth*
1 clove garlic, crushed

1 teaspoon salt
¼ teaspoon freshly ground pepper
½ teaspoon dried oregano
⅛ teaspoon paprika
2 onions, quartered
8 mushrooms
1 green pepper, cut into 8 squares

Cut meat into 1-inch cubes. Combine vinegar, oil, broth, garlic, and seasonings in bowl. Add meat and toss to coat all sides. Arrange meat alternately with vegetables on 4 skewers. Broil close to heat until meat is browned but still pink in the middle, about 12 minutes, turning often and brushing with marinade for moistness. *Makes 4 servings, 231 calories per serving.*

D.D. LONDON BROIL

1 teaspoon oil
2 teaspoons vinegar
2 tablespoons fat-free low-sodium bouillon
¼ teaspoon ground cloves

⅛ teaspoon freshly ground pepper
¼ teaspoon dried rosemary
1 clove garlic, mashed
1 flank steak or lean shoulder steak (about 1 pound)

Blend oil, vinegar, bouillon, and seasonings. Pierce flank steak with fork, then spread lightly with seasoning combination to coat all sides. Let stand a few minutes. Preheat broiler. Broil 4 inches from

(cont.)

heat for 5 minutes. Turn, brush with any remaining seasoning mixture, and brown other side 4 minutes. Steak should be pink in the middle; do not overcook. Cut into very thin diagonal slices to serve. (Any leftovers are delicious cold, for salad or open sandwiches.) *Makes 4 servings, 192 calories per serving.*

D.D. GREEN PEPPER STEAK

*½ pound round steak, ¼ inch
   thick, fat trimmed
1 tablespoon soy sauce*

*1 green pepper, cut into strips
1 cup nonfat low-sodium broth
1 cup precooked rice*

Cut steaks into strips about 2 inches long and 1 inch wide. Toss with soy sauce. Brown meat strips on one side in hot nonstick pan. Add green pepper strips and brown with meat, turning to cook both sides. Add broth and rice; stir and cook until pepper strips are tender and rice is hot, about 3 minutes. Cover and let stand 2 minutes more. *Makes 2 servings, 320 calories per serving.*

D.D. LAMB CHOPS ITALIENNE

*1 lean shoulder lamb chop (4 oz.)
2 tablespoons D.D. Italian
   Dressing*

Chopped parsley

Trim excess fat from lamb chop. Turn chop in Italian dressing to coat. Brown quickly in hot, ridged pan or on griddle or under broiler for about 5 minutes on each side. *1 serving at 244 calories.*

12

Delicious, Nutritious Key Recipes for Quick-Trim Diets and D.D. Nutri-Maintenance Eating

Here you'll find a unique and most helpful assortment of *key recipes* for use in the Delicious Basic and Variety Quick-Trim Diets, for Nutri-Maintenance Eating—and for all nutritious, flavorful, and satisfying food preparations from now on. You can make large quantities of these key recipes, if you like, and store them in the refrigerator or freezer for future use.

First, please review the D.D. Guidelines again in Chapter 9, and you're all set to cook up delicious D.D. treats. As stated a number of times for clarification, Delicious Diet Recipes—high in taste gratification while low in calories—are created to help you slim down and stay trim most enjoyably—if you like to cook. You may use them part of the time, all of the time, or not at all.

For example, where fish is specified in a meal, you may choose one of the Delicious Diet fish recipes, such as D.D. Halibut Florentine, or any available fish broiled or cooked any way you prefer within D.D. Guidelines. The same is true for vegetables, fruits, desserts, and other listed Basic Diet and/or Variety Diet servings.

All D.D. recipes have been carefully created, prepared, and tested for your maximum eating pleasure as well as for healthful reducing the Quick-Trim way. Preparation is clear and simple— there are no complicated instructions. Ingredients are readily obtainable; alternates are given for seasonal products you might not find year round. Because emphasis is on delicious, seasonal produce, and on poultry and fish (including inexpensive varieties), you may find that you save money, particularly on costly meat purchases.

As with all D.D. servings . . . *enjoy!*

D.D. VEGETABLE BROTH OR SOUP

D.D. Vegetable Broth or Soup is, unlike most broths, low in sodium, because it does not rely on salt, HVP (hydrolyzed vegetable protein), or monosodium glutamate for flavor. There are many prepared broths on the market (some low-sodium "instants" are available) but they lack D.D.'s full-broth satisfying flavor. The good taste and sweetness of D.D. Vegetable Broth comes from the vegetables used, and you can vary these to your taste as you become accustomed to making the broth.

You can also eat freshly made D.D. Vegetable Broth as a soup, with some of the fiber-rich vegetables included. Strain the broth and keep it in the refrigerator (or make a double batch and freeze some) to use as a "free" drink you can enjoy when you want it. There's no need to consider calories, since they are minimal.

D.D. Vegetable Broth also provides a flavorful cooking base for many dishes. Unlike broths made with meat or poultry, this is entirely fat free, needs no skimming, and is ready in a fraction of the time.

As you can see, there are a number of ingredients in this broth. If you wish to eliminate some, do so to your taste. We suggest that you make at least this sizable quantity, or more, since the broth is so useful and nutritious. If you want to keep it longer than 4 or 5 days (fine for refrigerator storage), pour the remainder into convenient-sized containers and freeze.

2 medium onions, chopped (about 1 cup)

2 cups chopped celery with tops, (4 to 5 stalks) or 2 cups chopped zucchini

1 cup coarsely cut spinach (or cabbage or broccoli leaves or escarole lettuce)

2 cups chopped or sliced carrots

¼ cup chopped flat (Italian) parsley (more flavorful than curly)

1 large clove garlic, peeled

¼ teaspoon crushed red pepper or ⅛ teaspoon ground red pepper

2 bay leaves

1½ quarts water

2½ cups tomato juice or canned tomatoes

2 tablespoons chopped fresh basil or 2 teaspoons dried

1 tablespoon chopped fresh thyme or 1 teaspoon dried

¾ teaspoon salt (optional)

(cont.)

Combine chopped vegetables, parsley, garlic, pepper, bay leaves, water, and tomato juice in a large saucepan. Simmer, covered, 30 minutes. Add basil, thyme, and salt if desired. Cook 10 minutes longer. Serve hot as soup, or strain through a fine sieve and chill as broth to have as wanted, hot or cold, or to use in cooking. *Makes about 1½ quarts broth.*

D.D. CHICKEN BROTH

Prepared "instant" chicken soup generally has no fat—but it is also usually high in sodium. Canned chicken broth with fat may be chilled, and fat removed as below.

"Stockpile" chicken parts as you prepare chicken for your meals: wrap in freezer wrap and store in freezer for homemade "bonus" soup stock.

4 pounds chicken bones and trimmings (wings, necks, gizzards, backs)
3 quarts cold water
1 teaspoon salt
8 white peppercorns

1 onion, peeled and studded with 3 cloves
2 carrots, peeled and sliced
1 herb bouquet (celery tops, parsley, fresh dill, and a bay leaf, tied together)

Cover chicken parts and bones with water. Add salt and peppercorns. Bring to a boil, then reduce heat and simmer 30 minutes. Skim. Add onion and carrots, cover, and simmer about 1½ hours. Add herb bouquet and simmer 30 minutes longer. Strain stock through fine sieve or cheesecloth; let cool at room temperature, then chill. Fat will rise to the surface, making it easy to remove. *Makes about 2 quarts chicken broth.*

D.D. FISH STOCK

3 pounds fish scraps, bones, and
   heads (split) or inexpensive
   whole fish
2 quarts water
4 stalks celery with tops, chopped

2 large onions, sliced
½ teaspoon dried thyme
5 sprigs parsley
1 bay leaf
Juice of 1 lemon

Tie fish scraps, bones, and head in cheesecloth, or place directly in stainless-steel or enameled pot with water and remaining ingredients. Bring to a boil, reduce the heat and simmer, partially covered, for about 25 minutes, then add the lemon juice.

Place pot in the kitchen sink, strain stock or lift out cheesecloth with bones, and hang the bag over the pot, allowing juices to drip back into pot. Gently squeeze the remaining liquid into the pot. Use as is, or boil the stock longer to reduce to 6 cups for well-flavored broth or poaching liquid. Use as a base for fish soups, stews, sauces, and to cook fish and seafood.

D.D. "CRÈME FRAÎCHE"

Note these calorie comparisons:
Heavy cream: Per tablespoon 52 calories, per cup 838 calories.
Low-fat yogurt: Per tablespoon 7.5 calories, per cup 120 calories.
Sour cream: Per tablespoon 29 calories, per cup 464 calories.
D.D. "Crème Fraîche": Per tablespoon 15 calories, per cup 210 calories.

⅞ cup plain low-fat yogurt

2 tablespoons heavy sweet cream

Combine yogurt and cream in container and stir smooth. (For lighter texture, greater volume, whip sweet cream before combining.) This

(cont.)

small amount of cream holds yogurt in smooth suspension. Use very sparingly as topping or ingredient in recipes. Even better if you refrigerate 24 hours to 4 days. To avoid temptation, store remainder of cream in the freezer until next use. Portion into small paper cups, 2 tablespoons each, for convenience. Defrost as needed, to stir with yogurt for more "crème fraîche." *Makes 1 cup.*

D.D. RICOTTA OR COTTAGE CRÈME

The "crème" can be used as is, instead of higher calorie cream, to bind or top dishes, or it can be flavored according to the dish it accompanies. Add a grating of lemon or orange rind, or cinnamon or a dash of vanilla or a liqueur, for a sauce for fresh fruit or fruit desserts. Or add a touch of savory seasoning, or caraway, or curry, or herbs to taste, and use to top soup and vegetables.

*½ cup skim milk ricotta or low-fat   ½ cup plain low-fat yogurt
    cottage cheese*

Puree cheese and yogurt in a blender or food processor until very smooth, or force cheese through a fine sieve, then beat well with yogurt. *Makes 1 cup, about 14 calories per tablespoon.*

WHITE CHEESE

Use only half the proportion of yogurt (for example, ½ cup cheese and ¼ cup yogurt) in the recipe above to make a soft smooth "white cheese," for spreading or cooking.

D.D. HERBED LOW-FAT COTTAGE CHEESE

¼ cup low-fat plain yogurt
8 ounces low-fat cottage cheese
1 tablespoon chopped fresh parsley

1 tablespoon chopped fresh chives
1 teaspoon dried tarragon

Combine all ingredients in blender container and blend until smooth, or mash and blend well with a fork. Empty cheese mixture into crock or small bowl. Chill to serve as wanted. *Makes about 1¼ cups; 44 calories per ¼ cup.*

D.D. CARAWAY COTTAGE CHEESE

In place of herbs in recipe above, add 1 tablespoon caraway seeds and 1 teaspoon grated orange rind.

D.D. MELTY MOZZARELLA APPETIZER

2 slices tomato
2 small slices mozzarella cheese
   (1 oz. total)

4 slivers red pepper
Basil
Lettuce leaves

Top tomato slices with mozzarella. Garnish with slivers of red pepper and sprinkle with basil. Broil or microwave until cheese is melty. Arrange on lettuce leaves. *Makes 2 servings, 45 calories each.*

D.D. "MAYO"

Use this as is or as an ingredient in recipes—or flavor with chopped chives, parsley, garlic, a pinch of chili or curry, or to your taste.

1 cup low-fat cottage cheese
1 egg
1 tablespoon vegetable oil

1 tablespoon lemon juice
Pinch each of mustard, paprika, salt, and cayenne

Combine all in bowl or food processor and beat until very smooth. *Makes 1½ cups at 14 calories per tablespoon (regular mayonnaise has 101 calories per tablespoon).*

D.D. ORANGE MAYO

Omit lemon juice in recipe above and replace with 1 tablespoon orange juice and 2 teaspoons grated orange rind.

D.D. GREEN GODDESS DRESSING

Add to *D.D. "Mayo" ingredients ¼ cup parsley, ¼ cup chopped spinach, 1 teaspoon dill, and 1 teaspoon anchovy paste (optional). Whirl in food processor or beat smooth. *Makes 1½ cups, 17 calories per tablespoon.*

D.D. CREAMY CUCUMBER DRESSING

*2 tablespoons *D.D. "Mayo" or low-calorie salad dressing*
2 tablespoons plain low-fat yogurt

2 tablespoons chopped, peeled cucumber
Salt, pepper, dill weed

(cont.)

Stir "mayo" and yogurt together until smooth. Add chopped cucumber, season to taste, and stir. Use on salad immediately; do not store. *Makes 6 tablespoons, 13 calories per tablespoon.*

D.D. FRENCH SALAD DRESSING

⅓ cup *D.D. Vegetable Broth or nonfat low-sodium vegetable broth or tomato juice
1 tablespoon wine vinegar (red or white)
1 tablespoon lemon juice

1 teaspoon vegetable oil
1 clove garlic, peeled and minced
Salt (optional) and freshly cracked black pepper
Pinch of dry mustard

Combine all ingredients in bowl and whisk with fork, or combine in a cruet, cover, and shake vigorously before each use. *Makes ⅔ cup dressing, 6 calories per tablespoon.*

D.D. ITALIAN SALAD DRESSING

Add to recipe above 1 slice onion or 1 scallion, finely minced (or 1 teaspoon instant minced onion), dash crushed red pepper. *6 calories per tablespoon.*

D.D. ZESTY TOMATO DRESSING

⅓ cup tomato juice
1 tablespoon wine vinegar
1 tablespoon lemon juice
1 teaspoon vegetable oil

1 clove garlic, minced
Pinch of dry mustard
Salt (optional)
Black pepper

Combine all ingredients in jar with tight-fitting lid; cover. Shake to blend before using. *Makes ⅔ cup, 6 calories per tablespoon.*

D.D. DILL DRESSING

Add to *D.D. French Dressing 1 teaspoon dried dill weed.

D.D. NON-OIL SALAD DRESSING

¼ teaspoon salt
¼ teaspoon paprika
¼ teaspoon mustard
¼ teaspoon freshly ground pepper
1 teaspoon chopped onion

1 teaspoon chopped fresh parsley
1 teaspoon chopped green pepper
½ cup *D.D. Vegetable Broth or
  tomato juice

Combine all ingredients in shaker-top jar; shake well and chill.
Makes about ½ cup dressing at 27 calories, 3 calories per tablespoon.

D.D. ORIENTAL SALAD DRESSING

1 teaspoon light soy sauce
2 tablespoons vinegar
2 tablespoons unsweetened
  applesauce

¼ teaspoon sesame oil or other oil
Dash ground ginger

Combine all ingredients. Stir with rice and/or stir-fried vegetables
to make salad. *Makes 2 servings, 20 calories per serving.*

D.D. HERB SEASONING MIX

1 teaspoon dried dill weed or
  celery seed
1 teaspoon dried basil or chopped
  fresh parsley

½ teaspoon paprika
¼ teaspoon garlic powder
⅛ teaspoon dried lemon peel
Pinch of mustard

(cont.)

Combine all ingredients in small bowl; mash to a powder and blend well. Store in a small plastic shaker. Vary to taste, combining sweet, sour, sharp, and mellow herbs and spices for a balance of flavors.

D.D. TOMATO SAUCE

3 pounds fresh ripe plum tomatoes
   or 1 can (1 pound, 12 ounces)
   Italian peeled tomatoes
½ cup water
1 small onion, peeled and finely
   minced
1 clove garlic, peeled and minced

1 rib celery, finely minced
2 tablespoons chopped parsley
2 tablespoons finely minced fresh
   basil or 2 teaspoons dried basil
1 sprig fresh thyme or ½ teaspoon
   dried thyme
Salt (optional) and pepper to taste

If fresh tomatoes are used, plunge into boiling water for half a minute. Cool under running water and slip off skins. For fresh or canned, cut away the stem ends and chop coarsely, reserving juices. Heat water in large nonstick skillet. Add onion, garlic, and celery and cook, stirring, until the vegetables are just tender, but not at all colored. Add tomatoes with their juices and bring to a boil; cook 10 minutes. Add parsley, basil, thyme, optional salt, and pepper. Simmer 10 minutes to thicken slightly. Cool to room temperature; then, if desired, store in screwtop jar in refrigerator for up to a week. *Makes 3½ cups, 26 calories per ¼-cup serving, 6 calories per tablespoon.*

D.D. HOLLANDAISE SAUCE

1 egg
1 tablespoon white wine vinegar
   or raspberry vinegar
3 tablespoons *D.D. Chicken
   Broth or nonfat low-sodium
   chicken broth

1 teaspoon lemon juice
1 tablespoon sweet butter, softened
Pinch each of cayenne, salt, dry
   mustard

(cont.)

Place all ingredients in double boiler over simmering water and beat with a wire whisk until thick and creamy. *Makes ½ cup, 24 calories per tablespoon.*

D.D. SALSA

The spicy sauce of Mexico, used as a condiment for simply broiled or steamed foods, as a seasoning for salads, or as an ingredient for dishes such as *D.D. Eggplant Mexicali, offers delicious and satisfying zesty flavor, as hot as you want it—and with few calories. The coriander used may be called "cilantro" in your market, or "Chinese parsley." If you cannot find it, substitute parsley, although the flavor is not quite the same. It is simple to sprout coriander, from the seeds in a spice jar, right on your windowsill.

This recipe is moderately spicy; if you prefer *mild*, substitute sweet green pepper for chilies.

¾ cup freshly cooked or canned round tomatoes, finely chopped
1 medium white onion, finely chopped

2 sprigs coriander, leaves only, finely chopped
3 to 4 fresh or canned hot green chilies, finely chopped
⅓ cup cold water

Chop the ingredients for this sauce with a knife, not in a processor or blender, in order to retain some texture in the sauce. Combine all ingredients and serve. Store remainder in refrigerator, covered. Keeps about 2 weeks—but you are likely to use it up sooner. Stir before serving. *Makes 1½ cups, 53 calories per cup, 3 calories per tablespoon.*

13

Extra-Quick Reducing Aids: *Delicious 3-Day Vegetable Diet and *Delicious 1-Day _____Liquid Diet—

with Special Delicious Recipes . . .

There's no question that the great majority of overweights on the Delicious Quick-Trim Diet lose weight rapidly, and keep taking it off, until they are down to their desired goal and trimmed to their most attractive personal dimensions. The D.D. calories-IN calories-OUT balance assures that.

While they are delighted with their weight-loss results, some individuals at times want to reduce even more speedily. Furthermore, after a week or two of rapid weight loss, some people may reach what is generally labeled a "plateau." They state that, after losing up to a pound or more per day for a period of time, they either lose weight more slowly or appear to remain stable. If this happens, they become concerned, since they want to keep reducing more quickly.

If *you* reach a "plateau," or want to take off pounds more rapidly, here are simple, effective steps you can take:

1. *Stay on your Delicious Diet,* and be doubly sure that you don't deviate from the D.D. Guidelines. You may have let up a little, or even a lot, without realizing it, as many people do. They gradually eat more, adding a high-calorie dish here and a rich, sauced dessert and a sugared snack there. So please reread the D.D. Guidelines, and stay within them exactly.

Realize too, as noted earlier, that the more overweight a person is, the faster he or she will lose weight. As you shed more pounds, you have less excess fat to take off. Naturally, the amount of daily loss in weight diminishes.

Just stay on the diet faithfully. Those individuals who reach a leveling off find that, after a few days of adhering to D.D. precisely, they enjoy a sudden drop of several pounds, sometimes overnight. Thereafter they continue to lose excess weight steadily.

2. *Cut down on the size of the portions you consume.* You may be taking in more food than at the start of your dieting, more than you need, again without being aware of eating more. It's simple arithmetic that if you overeat even low-calorie dishes, they'll add up to more calories consumed daily than your body uses up. As a result, you gain pounds and inches instead of losing them.

I ran into a D.D. dieter at a wedding recently as she was returning from the buffet table. She looked down at her huge, overflowing plate, reddened, and said hurriedly, "Look, they're all D.D.-permitted foods. . . ." I didn't say a word. She murmured, "I'm going to eat only half of this anyway." A week before she'd complained that the diet wasn't working rapidly enough for her.

3. *Be more watchful and reduce your salt intake even further without becoming extremist about it.* Switch to low-sodium foods wherever possible. Check salt/sodium content of packaged foods when you shop—*before* you buy. Servings high in salt tend to increase water retention, adding to your weight and to body bloat. Inflation (body inflation, that is) may be linked to high salt intake in many instances.

4. *Check with your doctor about water retention.* Upon reexamination and testing, regardless of what you eat, your physician may find that you need a diuretic (usually a small pill, or other medication) to combat excess water retention and to increase the volume of urine you excrete. Your blood pressure and other bodily functions keep changing with time. Don't assume that a diuretic is not needed because it hasn't been prescribed previously; check and be sure.

5. *Increase your level of activity, whatever your choice of physical conditioning may be* (see our recommendations in Chapter 17). If, for example, you are now walking briskly for fifteen continuous minutes daily, try to extend that period to twenty minutes or half an hour.

Proper activity is an excellent conditioning and health aid, *but is not effective enough alone as a reducing program.* It all hinges on the calories-IN calories-OUT governing equation. Stepping up your activity may help to speed up your rate of weight loss, especially if you have been sedentary—that is, too much sitting and lying about, and too little physical exertion.

144

DELICIOUS 3-DAY VEGETABLE EATING

As a change of pace, it has been found that some dieters whose rate of losing weight has slowed down can break the plateau barrier by switching to vegetable eating for a few days. That's *vegetable* eating, not "vegetarian." It's important to make that distinction, since there are dozens of different types of "vegetarians," some of whom have no interest in losing weight.

Among those vegetarians who eat vegetables *plus* vegetable oils and heavy dressing, breads in unlimited quantity, cakes, pudding, sugar, honey, syrups, lots of nuts, whole milk and cream, butter, margarine, eggs, and so on—many are overweight. As a vegetarian, you could pile in thousands of calories per day with that range of food in sizable portions.

On the other hand, you could eat just about as much as you want of the low-calorie vegetables (only a few are high calorie, as listed later)—just the vegetables themselves—and you'll probably never become overweight. Many adults who eat that way may be healthy, vigorous, and trim year after year.

This kind of all-vegetable consumption is not advisable for the growing youngster, even into the later teens, despite claims otherwise by some vegetarians. Furthermore, annual medical checkups are desirable for adult vegetarians, as for all other individuals.

However, your concern here, and ours, is that of switching to vegetables for a very limited time, in order to combat any plateau standstill, or for a few days of extra-quick weight loss. You'll be aided by a vital change in types of foods consumed, and you'll be cutting intake to about 600 calories per day. Try it and see the weight drop for yourself.

DELICIOUS 3-DAY VEGETABLE DIET

Observe these guidelines:

1. This diet is for three days only—so return to your D.D. Basic Diet or D.D. Variety Diet after the three days. No, it's not "dangerous" for the person in normal health to continue this diet for a week or two, or even more if still overweight. We prefer, however, to set the three-day limitation, since that period should accomplish your purpose. Please get your doctor's permission (a phone call should do it) to eat just vegetables for the brief period.

The very special feature of this diet, making it different and superior to any other vegetarian eating, is that you'll enjoy your meals exceptionally with tasteful and satisfying D.D. Vegetable Recipes. You can delight in them at every meal, if you like to cook.

Also, check the additional taste tips in Chapter 16, which apply here. They can help you get increased enjoyment from the enhanced flavor of each serving. The D.D. all-important *extra* applies here too: Lift the taste factor without elevating the calorie content.

2. *Eat moderate portions of any four vegetables in the following list, three times daily.* (Vegetables may be cooked or raw in many instances, as you prefer.) Or you may have a plateful of *three vegetables four times daily*—or servings *of two vegetables six times a day*—as you please, your personal choice:

Artichokes—whole, hearts	Lettuce—all types
Arugula (rugula, rocket salad)	Mushrooms
Asparagus	Okra
Bamboo shoots	Onions
Bean sprouts	Parsley*
Beans—green, wax	Peppers
Broccoli	Potatoes**
Cabbage—regular, Chinese	Radishes
Carrots	Sauerkraut
Cauliflower	Spinach
Celery	Summer squash
Chives*	Tomatoes
Cucumbers	Tomato juice***
Eggplant	Turnips
Endive	Vegetable juice***
Kale	Watercress
Kohlrabi	

*These and other herbs are permitted.

**Enjoy a medium-size plain baked, boiled, or mashed potato—no more than one daily—if you wish. Instead of the potato once daily, you may substitute ½ cupful of boiled rice or pasta (macaroni, spaghetti, noodles), no fats or sauces added; use herbs, spices, or other seasoning, and a D.D. dressing or bottled low-calorie dressing, to your taste.

***Tomato juice or vegetable juice (no sugar added) may be substituted for a vegetable, if desired, although the vegetable is more filling due to greater bulk.

NOT PERMITTED: The following fine vegetables are higher in calories than those on the preceding list, and are to be avoided while you're on the diet:

Avocados	Peas
Beans—lima, red kidney	Pumpkin
Beets	Soybeans
Corn	Sweet potatoes, yams
Lentils	Winter squash

    For Nutri-Maintenance Eating later, keep in mind that pumpkin and winter squash, while higher than summer squash, are lower than carbohydrate alternatives such as rice or pasta. Even high-calorie avocado can be enjoyed later as *D.D. Guacamole—a spread lower in calories than butter.

    3. *Cook the vegetables as you please, within D.D. Guidelines (no fats, no sugar, limited use of salt)—using the delectable D.D. recipes for vegetables and salads; use recipes of your own, or as served in eating out (no added fats, heavy sauces, or dressings, of course)—again* your personal choice.

    Make up your menus for three meals a day, or divided into four, five, or six meals during the day. Here's an example:

    Breakfast: Vegetable juice and a hot vegetable such as *D.D. Baked Nutmeg Apple Summer Squash, or another favorite D.D. recipe. Coffee.

    Lunch: Tomato juice and your choice of three vegetables, or a large combination salad, or another salad. Tea or coffee or another permitted beverage such as no-sugar ginger ale.

    Dinner: *D.D. Asparagus Velvet Soup, and two vegetables (don't forget delectable D.D. recipes), along with a sizable salad with a D.D. dressing or other low-calorie dressing, lemon juice, or herbed vinegar. Coffee, tea (why not try one of the D.D. coffee or tea recipes?), or another permitted beverage.

    If wanted, between meals you may enjoy permitted snacks, and no-calorie beverages at any time.

    The Delicious Three-Day Vegetable Diet is simple, satisfying, and effective for extra weight loss. You'll be consuming lots of food, will feel full, yet the whole quantity is low in total calories. You can't help but lose weight rapidly on this three-day diet if you follow D.D. Guidelines correctly, since you'll be eating an average of about 600 calories daily.

4. *Enjoy as snacks any time any of the permitted vegetables raw*— dipped into one of the D.D. seasoned dips, if you like. You may also have between meals—up to three cups daily—a cup of low-calorie, low-sodium onion or vegetable instant broth, or *D.D. Vegetable Broth—filling, satisfying, and a delicious asset for desired weight control.

5. *Drink lots of no-calorie liquids.* That includes water, seltzer, no-salt-added club soda, coffee (preferably decaffeinated), teas— herb teas and no-sugar flavored teas—sugar-free carbonated beverages. You may have a dash of skim milk in coffee or tea—or a squeeze of lemon in tea is fine—but no sugar (artificial sweetener is permitted, but don't overload).

6. *Don't add butter, margarine, oil, mayonnaise, or any other rich dressing, or any high-calorie ingredients to the vegetables.* If you do, you'll defeat the purpose of this diet, which is to provide a change of pace from the two primary Delicious Diets—and to reduce your daily intake to an average of about 600 calories.

7. *Don't eat bread, cakes, cookies, candies, ice cream, puddings, other high-calorie sweets and desserts.* If you deviate, you'll be negating the swift slimming action of this diet.

8. *Don't eat anything that is not listed as permitted while on this diet.* As one example, don't eat nuts—nutritious but high in calories. You'll be able to enjoy them and other favorites once you're down to your wanted weight, and in very limited amounts on the Delicious Basic and Variety Diets.

9. *Don't have any alcoholic drinks while on the Delicious Three-Day Vegetable Diet.* You may have such drinks, within the limitations specified, when you return to other D.D. dieting and eating.

10. *Skip any meal if you wish.* Once you feel that you've had enough, or simply don't care for any more food, it's smart to stop eating at that time. Just keep drinking plenty of the permitted liquids.

11. *Have a vitamin-mineral capsule daily* if you care to, but it's not essential.

12. *Don't overeat at any one time.* This is more a matter of good bodily functioning and good health rather than concern about excess calories.

13. *Stop dieting if you don't feel well.* There is rarely any reason

for not feeling good when dieting for only three days at a time on these nutritious vegetables, but don't take any chances. If you start to feel weak or ill in any way, *stop*. Return to regular dieting and eating until you feel well. If you have any further concern at all, check with your doctor. This Delicious Three-Day Vegetable Diet, like others in this book, is for adults, not for growing youngsters.

14. *When you eat out in restaurants or homes, choose from whatever D.D. vegetables are available,* keeping within the D.D. Guidelines as much as possible (again, don't get uptight about it). In someone else's home, just eat whatever vegetables and salad are being served, avoiding added fats, dressings, and sauces as much as you can. In restaurants, order available vegetables of your choice, asking that they be prepared and served plain with no added fats, dressings, or sauces. Specify whatever salad you choose "without dressing."

Ask for lemon wedges so you can squeeze fresh lemon juice on vegetables for extra flavor. Also request vinegar, if you like it, for salads. If you've prepared *D.D. Herb Seasoning Mix, carry some with you to sparkle up vegetables and salads when eating out as well as at home.

15. *Check your weight on the scale chart first thing every morning.* Mark down each day's number of pounds on the D.D. scale chart. You'll get the extra incentive of seeing the pounds drop off day after day.

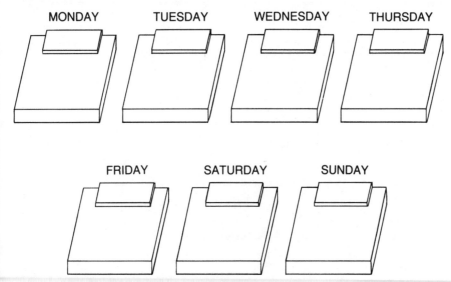

MONDAY   TUESDAY   WEDNESDAY   THURSDAY

FRIDAY   SATURDAY   SUNDAY

D.D. THREE-DAY VEGETABLE DIET MENUS

As with all Delicious Diets, use the D.D. vegetable recipes or your own choice of vegetables, at home or eating out, within D.D. Guidelines.

DAY ONE

Breakfast

*D.D. Fresh Carrot-Lemon Drink
*D.D. Oatmeal with Grated Apple
Herb tea *or* *D.D. Uncoffee au Lait

Midmorning snack

*D.D. Vegetable Broth (warm or cold) *or* low-sodium vegetable-tomato juice *or* carrot sticks

Lunch

Large green salad with lettuce, celery, spinach leaves, shredded carrots, alfalfa sprouts, and pumpkin seeds
*D.D. Green Goddess Dressing
Two jícama slices (or zucchini spears) for munching

Afternoon snack

*D.D. Gazpacho (6 ounces)

Dinner

*D.D. Artichoke Vinaigrette *or* *D.D. Vegetable Melange in Foil *or* *D.D. Gingered Stir-Fry Vegetables with Chicken or Turkey (leaving out the chicken or turkey)
*D.D. Uncooked Applesauce

Night snack

*D.D. Vegetable Broth (warm or cold)

DAY TWO

Breakfast

Apple juice with lemon wedge
Cottage cheese with cinnamon and granulated sugar substitute
Herb tea *or* *D.D. Uncoffee au Lait

Midmorning snack

Celery sticks and *D.D. Herbed Low-Fat Cottage Cheese

Lunch

*D.D. Health Salad
*D.D. French *or* Italian Salad Dressing

Dinner

*D.D. Pasta Primavera
*D.D. Mandarin Orange Sections
Tea *or* *D.D. Espresso Coffee

Night Snack

Seltzer with orange wedge

DAY THREE

Breakfast

½ cantaloupe with lemon wedge
Cottage cheese with grated carrot and Grape-Nuts
Herb tea *or* hot apple juice

Midmorning Snack

Cherry tomatoes

Lunch

1 cup *D.D. Eggplant-Zucchini Salad, chilled, with *D.D. Marinated Mushrooms and rice
Apple wedges
Tea *or* coffee

Afternoon Snack

*D.D. Vegetable Broth (warm or cold)

Dinner

*D.D. Steamed Vegetable Platter
Sliced banana with pineapple juice
Spiced Tea *or* *D.D. Slim Cappuccino

Night Snack

Seltzer with lemon wedge

Another way to speed up weight loss, and also to overcome a plateau stalemate, is the ultra-simple Delicious One-Day Liquid Diet. If you wish, you may use it any one day of the week. What makes this D.D. system so different from any other liquid diet is that you enjoy the special Delicious Liquid Diet Drink. Easy to prepare, it's a refreshing lift and energy boost while on your Delicious One-Day Liquid Diet—and any time you wish to enjoy it thereafter.

Some people like to go on this diet once every week. They report that they not only drop more pounds by the next day, but that they also feel "cleansed," a sense of relief throughout the body. They declare enthusiastically that any discomfort they'd encountered before the day of liquid dieting, being bloated and overfull because of overweight, was greatly relieved due to drinking the permitted liquids only on the Liquid Diet.

They also affirm that after being on the Delicious One-Day Liquid Diet, rather than having any sense of weakness or dizziness—as might be expected by the inexperienced—*they enjoy an upsurge of special well-being, even exhilaration.*

Many like to go on the diet every Monday, after the weekend's eating. That's fine for one day a week—whatever day you choose is okay. In the great majority of cases, however, the regular Delicious Basic or Variety Diets will bring down your weight quickly and beautifully without your ever using the Liquid Diet.

Before you undertake even one day of no-food dieting, you should phone your doctor to get the go-ahead. Some individuals become very concerned about skipping a single meal, let alone not eating for a day. But for people in normal health, this is a groundless fear, since the body survives well by feeding on its own fat, as has been pointed out before.

There are countless instances of people surviving for lengthy periods without solid food, but not without liquid. In a highly publicized incident some years back, a man and woman in a small airplane crashed in the Yukon wilderness. In the first few days they used up all of the very small amount of food they'd brought aboard for the expected brief flight. Aggravating their problems, the man had sustained cracked ribs and a broken jaw in the accident. Temperatures in the ice- and snow-covered area were as low as 45 degrees below zero.

With all food gone, the two people kept themselves alive with melted snow as their only liquid and sustenance. Finally they were rescued, *forty-nine days after they'd crashed.* After being cared for in a hospital, they went through extensive medical examinations. The result: Neither of them, it was reported, had suffered any detectable lasting organic damage, in spite of weeks without food and considerable loss of weight.

No, we definitely don't recommend this kind of physical and emotional ordeal as a method for taking off weight. Two less hardy individuals might not have survived. The facts are simply illustrative of what the human body can accommodate at times on a very limited or strictly liquid diet.

Nor do we recommend fasting for more than a day or two unless specified by a physician, and then you should be monitored regularly by trained personnel. For obese patients who are 50 or even 100 or more pounds above average weight for their height, a number of hospitals have established effective starvation programs. Some of these courses run from three weeks to four months, usually under daily supervision.

With the overwhelming majority of patients, these formerly obese women and men emerged from the hospitals much trimmer and with remarkably improved health. They had a far better chance for a more vigorous, longer life. It must be stressed that these hospital starvation programs are for cases of extreme overweight, definitely not for the person with fewer than fifty pounds to lose.

In practically all cases of this kind of fasting, by substituting liquids for solid foods a good deal of the time, the dieters report that soon after they started the program, they didn't feel ravenously hungry, nor did they have an increased craving for food. Many said happily that as their appetites diminished, they felt comfortable, even invigorated.

A significant factor was that drinking lots of liquid helped keep them feeling "full" rather than "empty." That's true also with the Delicious One-Day Liquid Diet. Another supportive point for you is that the ex-patients didn't have any compulsion to eat larger quantities of food on the days following their shift from liquid dieting to an average diet.

After digesting the details that follow, decide for yourself whether or not you wish to consider trying the One-Day Liquid Diet.

You needn't be concerned about what food to eat and what not to eat on this diet because for the one day you don't eat any-thing—aside from the permitted liquids that you drink. From this clear viewpoint, there could hardly be an easier diet. However, you must follow these instructions and precautions precisely:

1. *Phone your doctor before starting,* just to make sure that you have no condition that would keep you from going on this liquid regimen for a day. If your physician has any doubts, don't proceed.

2. *Enjoy the special Delicious Liquid-Diet Drink*—which you prepare as a "quart-a-day" in orange or apple flavor, to sip for three "meals" and a snack. The quick, easy recipe is included here, as well as a choice of beverages.

3. *Drink 8 or more glasses of water during your waking hours.* That may sound like a lot until you realize that it's *less than half a glass an hour* for every hour awake during the 24-hour day. (It's a plus that drinking plenty of water is considered a fine skin aid—ask your dermatologist.)

4. *As alternatives, drink as much as you want of the following beverages, your personal choice.* You don't have to drink all or any, but be sure you get plenty of liquid, even if you prefer to stay with plain water (tap or bottled water is okay):

- *Hot or iced coffee* (preferably decaffeinated), now available in many blends. Yes, you may have espresso, if you like—no sugar, but a piece of lemon peel afloat is fine.
- Hot or iced tea (decaffeinated now available) . . . many delicious varieties in regular teas.
- Hot or iced packages of no-sugar "herb teas" in a variety of flavors. We recommend that you use packaged brands of such teas, prepared by knowledgeable people. Amateurs sometimes unknowingly use dangerous ingredients in making their own "herb" concoctions.
- Carbonated beverages, artificially sweetened, no sugar, as many glasses as wanted in reasonable quantity, during the Liquid Diet day.

5. *No sugar, milk, or cream should be added to any of the liquids during the Liquid Diet day.*

6. *Artificial sweetener and a squeeze of fresh lemon or lime* may be added to any of the liquids and beverages, as you please, but avoid excess use.

7. *No solid food is to be eaten while on the One-Day Liquid Diet.*

Drinking only the liquids and beverages permitted, you'll be consuming practically no significant calories for the one day.

8. *Proceed with normal activity during the entire diet day*—walking, moving about, working. If your work is very strenuous, save this diet for a weekend day. Avoid more demanding exertions such as running, jogging, vigorous bicycling and calisthenics, swimming, and other sports. Although usually such activity is recommended as part of your regular D.D. Program (but never in excess), skip it while on the One-Day Liquid Diet. Also, put off any very strenuous outdoor work such as digging a new garden area, shoveling snow, or heavy indoor housecleaning (don't you like *that* dieting restriction?).

9. *Avoid other more exhausting pursuits for the day.* For example, it's not desirable to have a sauna, steam bath, very hot water bath or shower, or to endure lengthy sunbathing.

10. *Definitely skip alcoholic drinks and smoking for the Liquid Diet day* (if you're a heavy smoker who can't manage without cigarettes, cut down to fewer than six this day).

11. *Take a therapeutic vitamin-mineral capsule* this day with one of the beverages.

12. *Go off the diet at once if you feel ill in any way, queasy, faint, or weak*—which should not occur during a one-day abstinence from solid food—and return to your regular Delicious Diet. Don't take any chances—feeling good is more important than losing weight.

13. *Partnership tip:* You may find it helpful, as a sort of competitive game, to undertake the limited-time Vegetable or Liquid diets with your husband or wife, a friend, another adult in the family, or an office acquaintance. You can compare experiences and give each other support.

AFTER THE ONE-DAY LIQUID DIET

In addition to the benefits already mentioned, those who have elected to go on the Liquid Diet once, or one day a week, state that they have been extremely impressed with the fact that they lost convincingly by cutting out solid food for the brief period. This proved to them again that their excess weight was due to *consuming too many calories,* and was not caused by any personal metabolic disorder or other abnormality.

Furthermore, going without solid food for a day demonstrated to them that they had the *willpower* to change their past overweight eating habits in order to lose weight. After a day on the Liquid Diet, they say it was a cinch to move on to the Delicious Quick-Trim Diet—without feeling deprived in any way.

Most important, they acquired additional assurance that they'd be able finally to stay trim always. One sighed with heartfelt relief and said the sustaining words: *"Never heavy again!"*

After your Delicious Three-Day Vegetable Diet, or your Delicious One-Day Liquid Diet (if you decide to try them), return to your regular Delicious Quick-Trim Diet if you have more pounds to lose before reaching your goal. If you're down to your desired weight, go on to Delicious Nutri-Maintenance Eating, as detailed in Chapter 15.

DELICIOUS ORANGE LIQUID-DIET DRINK

Make this great shake and divide it during the day, to your taste. Have one glass for breakfast, one for lunch; blend with ice cubes for a frothy dinner shake.

1½ cups instant nonfat dry milk solids	1 egg
3 cups cold water	¼ cup quick-cooking oats
1 can (6 ounces) frozen orange juice concentrate	2 teaspoons vanilla

Combine 1½ cups of the water and the remaining ingredients in blender. Blend on high for 30 seconds. Pour into a 2-quart container. Add remaining 1½ cups water and stir vigorously. Store in refrigerator to use throughout the day. Stir before each use. *Makes 4 generous 11 oz. servings, 218 calories each.*

DELICIOUS APPLE LIQUID-DIET DRINK

Substitute apple juice concentrate for the orange and ½ teaspoon ground cinnamon for the vanilla.

ONE-DAY LIQUID VARIETY DIET MENU

A menu for super-speedy weight loss, to sip with pleasure and variety through the day.

Breakfast

*D.D. Orange, Peach, or Strawberry "Instant" Breakfast
Coffee *or* tea

Midmorning Snack

*D.D. Vegetable Broth (warm or cold) *or* grapefruit juice *or* *D.D. Coffee Slim

Lunch

*D.D. Banana *or* Peach Shake

Afternoon Snack

Apple juice (6 ounces)

Dinner

*D.D. Curried Tuna Bisque
2 whole-wheat crispbread wafers (optional)

Night Snack

*D.D. Almond Skim-Milk Shake

14

How to Eat Out and Reduce ___Deliciously

It's just about as easy and effective to lose weight on the Delicious Quick-Trim Diet when you're eating out as at home. Of course, you won't be eating the exact D.D. recipes out, unless your hostess or restaurant chefs use them on their own. We expect that many restaurants, as well as fine home cooks, will be featuring D.D. recipes, listed right on restaurant menus.

However, most of the time *you simply follow the simple D.D. guidelines* in choosing what you eat out, precisely as you do at home whenever you don't prepare dishes from D.D. recipes.

EATING IN SOMEONE ELSE'S HOME

Specifically, when eating at someone else's home, if your hostess is serving a chicken dish (or if you choose chicken from a restaurant menu), you eat it in the most fat-free way possible—without being too obvious or fanatical about it. If the chicken is served with a heavy sauce, remove it discreetly (push the sauce to the side of your plate, along with any skin or visible fat) before eating your portion.

If the chicken (or other food) is richly oiled, or doused with thick gravy, just take a very small portion. Skip some of the side dishes if they are clearly highly caloric, without being obvious or offensive. By applying good sense and good taste, you can certainly handle the situation pleasantly.

No considerate hostess should protest if you say, "I've become a small eater—I look and feel better that way." Or if you turn down dessert, for example, explaining with a smile, "It looks wonderful, but I'm taking off weight and have to skip it for now. I'd love to enjoy it when I'm sylphlike."

If the hostess presses you, *she* is displaying a lack of consideration. Stick to your fundamental D.D. Guidelines without going overboard about it. Your attractive appearance and improved health are the most vital factors here, not pleasing an insensitive hostess.

If drinks are being offered, instead of having a cocktail or highball, have a nonalcoholic drink such as club soda or salt-free seltzer (preferable to salted carbonated waters), including imported types. Add ice cubes and a chunk of lime—and you'll be sipping the refreshing "D.D. highball" without imbibing extra calories (looks exactly like a gin or vodka tonic).

If a dry wine is being served, and you enjoy wine, have an ounce or two if you like. Sip it slowly to make it last, as true wine experts do, never gulping down the contents of a glass. With a moderate drink of dry wine (never sweet wines or other alcoholic drinks until you're slim), you'll still remain within easy, sensible D.D. Guidelines, and will continue losing weight Deliciously. You can look forward to indulging if you wish after you're down to your desired weight, as you'll learn in Chapter 15 when you switch to D.D. Nutri-Maintenance Eating for the rest of your slim-trim lifetime.

EATING OUT IN RESTAURANTS

It's very simple but essential when dining out at restaurants to choose from the menu according to D.D. Guidelines. Whatever you have decided upon for that meal, ask that they serve your portion without heavy sauce, or with the sauce "on the side," so you can use a little or not.

If you choose a chicken dish that you're not sure about, such as "Chicken à la maison" (which could be almost any style), ask how it's prepared. If it sounds highly caloric, order broiled, boiled, or roasted chicken, not fried or sautéed in butter or oil (cooked in wine without added fat is fine). Always remove any skin or visible fat before eating.

Follow the same guidelines with fish, shellfish, or meat. If you've ordered steak, be sure to say ahead of time that you don't want it served with butter or any sauce, except "on the side." If the waiter claims that it's a "very light sauce," have it on the side regardless, so you can see and decide for yourself. Be firm about it.

Similarly, order vegetables without butter or rich sauces. Ask for the salad without dressing, with "dressing on the side," or served plain with vinegar and/or lemon wedges, which you can apply as your low calorie (or no calorie) dressing. If you like, add some of your personal seasoning to salad and other foods from a small amount of a mixture you carry with you—*D.D. Herb Seasoning Mix, for example.

Fresh-squeezed lemon accentuates foods particularly for those who omit added salt—it's an aid to weight reduction because it reduces water absorption and an aid to flavor because taste perceptions are close to those for salt on the tongue. And if you do want to add salt, that's readily available.

A simple and effective seasoning trick is to carry a compact, portable pepper mill, filled with peppercorns, to grate freshly as needed.

When dining in restaurants, beware of unclear words and phrases that may denote high-calorie food preparation. Listings with fancy or foreign names are not necessarily delicious at all, but can sometimes be heavy, greasy, unpleasantly and indigestibly rich. Examples are "herbed butter sauce," "au gratin" (too often heavy, with rich cheese added, rather than delicate and light), "sautéed, fried, deep-fried, pan-fried," "creamed," "pot pie" (often with a thick, greasy crust), "à la mode" (may be a tough-crusted pie topped with concealing ice cream and loaded with calories), and other familiar terms that add unneeded fatty ingredients.

If you don't know exactly what the dish comprises in the particular eating place, it's good sense as well as good taste to ask—that's a diner's privilege. If you prefer your fish broiled "dry" or with wine rather than done with butter, cream, or other high-calorie additives, say so—it's certainly acceptable form, even in the classiest restaurants.

"Take home" is another thoroughly admissible request, no matter how deluxe the dining place. The hypocrisy of a "doggie bag" is out—no need to use an often imaginary pet as an excuse. You've paid for the food, and it's a compliment to the chef (as stated by a leading maître d') that you want to take along uneaten food to enjoy at home the next day. This is confirmed by the owners of the prestigious Homestead Inn in Greenwich, Connecticut, and in restaurants everywhere.

Insist on Getting Low-Fat Servings

It's smart and essential to persist pleasantly in having your food prepared at restaurants in the D.D. way when possible, and it usually is. A gourmet friend who has dined in many of the finest places worldwide relates this illustrative incident at a luxurious French café on New York's fashionable East Side:

"I chose Dover sole from the elaborate menu. The patronizing maître d' asked, 'Would you prefer your Dover sole cooked in our rich butter sauce with a dash of wine or our splendid cream sauce with capers and shallots?'

"I said, 'Isn't the Dover sole fresh and of high quality?'

"He retorted, 'We have the best and freshest fish anywhere!'

"I asked gently, 'Then why cover up the natural flavor with butter or cream sauces? Can't I get it broiled in a little good dry wine, seasoned lightly with herbs and fresh lemon?'

" 'But of course,' he said, smiling with new respect. 'That is the best way. Yet most of our customers. . . .' He shrugged expressively."

Similarly, I dined at the famous Le Café Chambord at the peak of its popularity. A frequent guest who had dined there several times that week asked the maître d', "Pierre, can't I have something choice and plain, no sauces or dressings?"

He suggested and brought her broiled chicken livers, not on the menu, marvelously seasoned, which she acclaimed as one of the best dishes she'd ever enjoyed at the Chambord. Try the comparable recipe for *D.D. Seasoned Chicken Livers at the end of this chapter.

Never hesitate to discuss exactly how you want your food prepared—*before ordering*. Those in charge are in business to please you so that you'll keep coming back. Perhaps in days past you might have been labeled a "fusspot," but not in this more enlightened time. Now people who really value good food and good health know that low-fat eating (as instructed in D.D. Guidelines) makes good sense, which *is* good taste.

If only rich desserts are listed on the menu, ask for fresh fruit or skip the dessert, as many people do in any case. Or ask what's available although not on the printed menu. Usually you can be served fresh or unsugared fruit, low-calorie and deliciously re-freshing—fresh berries, sliced orange, a melon sparkled up with a squeeze of lemon wedge, unsugared fresh fruit cup. Don't let what's out of sight keep the possibilities out of your mind.

ENJOYING D.D. FOODS AT WORK

Airtight containers in a huge variety of types and sizes now make it a cinch to take along lunches to the office or factory—and to save over restaurant prices. Simply select each day from the many D.D. lunch dishes included in the book. One container can hold a mixed salad, and another one of the D.D. dressings, for example.

If refrigeration is available where you are, choose your D.D. lunch accordingly. Otherwise take something that keeps well on its own. The same is true for the D.D. beverages and snacks you like—no problem that can't be handled readily from the wide choice in the D.D. menus. You'll be losing weight deliciously whether at home or out.

MORE EATING-OUT TIPS

- Remove all visible fat from foods when eating out, as well as at home. No matter how tempting the skin looks on your serving of chicken, turkey, or fish, remove it before eating. Remove fat from steak, roast beef, and other meats. Consuming the fat would load on extra calories and could ruin your digestion. For proof, look at the fat you've taken off and see how it has congealed into a repulsive mass on your plate.

  In poultry dishes, duck and goose are poor choices because they're more fatty to start with. Also, various fats are often added in preparation, cooking, and serving. If these are favorites of yours, enjoy them occasionally later when you've moved on to D.D. Nutri-Maintenance Eating.

- If hors d'oeuvres are being served with drinks at a cocktail party or dinner, turn down everything that isn't within D.D. Guidelines. Keep in mind that you may indulge, within personal limitations, *after* you've slimmed down to your desired weight. A great plus then is that any appetite for rich, greasy, high-calorie food probably will have changed.

163

Skip such common high-calorie appetizers as bologna, salty prosciutto wrapped around cream cheese, deep-fried little potato pancakes, fatty and spicy smoked fish. Simply say "no, thanks" when the tray comes around. If you're concerned about offending anyone, realize that if you had a medical condition, such as an ulcer, which prohibited certain "delicacies," you wouldn't hesitate to refuse forbidden foods.

You can enjoy the raw vegetables (*crudités*), dipping them in a touch of sauce if wanted, but not loading a stalk of celery, for instance, as a carrier for a massive cargo of creamy dip. The calories are just as high whether you eat a fattening mixture on celery or by the tablespoonful. On the other hand, if a thoughtful hostess is serving a choice of delectable, low-calorie dips, you can take special pleasure in savoring the delicious flavor without consuming excess calories.

Remember—nobody can force you to eat what you don't want, or can pressure you into being heavy, if you respect yourself and maintain your determination to lose weight.

Typically, at a lavish cocktail party, I saw trays of fancy, high-calorie hors d'oeuvres coming around as regularly as luggage on an airport turntable. A heavy man nearby was grabbing and stuffing down the rich concoctions while his slim, beautiful wife refused them with a smile. He said to her, "You're a fool to pass up these gorgeous delicacies!" She smoothed her trim hips and answered, "That's the kind of fool I want to be."

• If you're at a buffet lunch or dinner, select carefully so that you choose permitted D.D. foods, as in the daily listings. Always pass up creamy dishes such as Chicken à la king, or tuna, salmon, shrimp, meat, or other salads that are pre-mixed with thick mayonnaise or other high-calorie ingredients.

• Never overload your plate, even with low-calorie foods. That's a sure temptation to overeat. You can always go back for more. And don't hesitate to leave food on your plate—better that it be discarded rather than stuffed into you, adding unwanted pounds and inches to your body, as well as over-taxing your digestive system.

• When alcoholic drinks, soda, or other high-calorie beverages are being served, it's a great help to always hold a glassful of something in your hand (as many reformed alcoholics do).

That helps two ways: the act of sipping along with others maintains the socializing rhythm, and nobody will keep urging you to "have a drink"—since you're already holding one.

You have plenty of choices—a tall glass of water with ice cubes, or a "*D.D. highball" (seltzer and chunk of lime or lemon), no-sugar soda in a variety of flavors, or another no-calorie beverage. If coffee or tea is available, that's acceptable too (without cream or sugar, of course).

... Bonus Recipe ...

D.D. SEASONED CHICKEN LIVERS

½ pound chicken livers
1 tablespoon chopped fresh sage
  leaves or 1 teaspoon dried sage

2 tablespoons *D.D. Italian Salad
  Dressing

Trim chicken livers and pierce each several times with tines of a fork to prevent popping. Season with sage and toss with dressing. Spread livers in ridged pan or on a ridged foil. Preheat broiler and broil about 5 inches from the heat about 5 minutes, or until browned, then turn and cook 2 minutes on second side, until browned but still pink in the center. Garnish with lemon wedge. Serve with *D.D. Broiled Tomato Half and *D.D. Broiled Potato Slices or *D.D. Onion-Stuffed Mushrooms. *Makes 2 servings, with calories for liver portion 152 per serving.*

3

HOW YOU MAINTAIN TRIMNESS LIFELONG —DELICIOUSLY

15

D.D. Nutri-Maintenance Eating: Your Program for Delicious, Nutritious, Lifelong Slim-Trim Control

Including D.D. Five-Pound Switch System and Nutri-Maintenance Recipes

The lessons you've learned in getting down to your desired weight through your Delicious Quick-Trim Diet should keep you trim for the rest of your life. You now know conclusively that *you can enjoy Delicious food and stay trim, too.* You're all set for a beautifully slim, healthier lifestyle now and "forever"—as you switch to Delicious, nutritious, well-balanced, and controlled D.D. Nutri-Maintenance Eating.

Latest and long-proven findings support the D.D. program strongly. One example at this writing: The National Academy of Sciences has just issued a new set of recommendations on diet and cancer. It made clear that while the relationship between diet and cancer has not been established specifically, certain general precepts emerge.

As noted in a *New York Times* editorial: "Fat is the food most closely associated with cancer. The committee's recommendations are: eat less fat; eat more fruit, vegetables and whole grains; minimize salt-cured and smoked foods; consume alcohol, if at all, in moderation."

The Delicious Diets and Nutri-Maintenance Eating conform to these basic guidelines—highly important to your potentially healthier and longer life. In no sense, however, are the Academy statements or D.D. precepts to be taken as a guarantee of good health—there are too many affecting human and individual variations. As the *Times* emphasizes, "The relationships between diet and cancer are fraught with uncertainties, fads and fallacies. But certain rough shapes are beginning to emerge from the fog." (More facts in this area are provided in Chapter 21.)

169

As a thinking individual, you decide for yourself. One thing for sure: You'll maintain a slim, trim figure when you adhere to D.D. Nutri-Maintenance Eating. The program embodies triple benefits for you: (1) satisfying, Delicious foods; (2) healthy weight control; (3) advancement of enduring well-being with reduced risk.

VARIETY IS THE SPICE AND SUSTENANCE OF D.D. NUTRI-MAINTENANCE EATING

Variety is a key word for healthful, nutritious maintenance eating, as agreed upon by most qualified physicians and Ph.D.s in the field. Dr. Nevin Scrimshaw, as head of nutrition and food science at Massachusetts Institute of Technology, points out:

> *Many Americans were taught the seven basic food groups that make up a balanced diet . . . but the number of food groups, whether down to a simplified four or broken into numerous subdivisions, is not important. The message one should get—the most important concept one must know—is variety.*

REDEFINING "DELICIOUS"

Getting maximum gratification in every way out of eating is based on an updated definition of "delicious." First, a dictionary definition:
> de·li·cious (dĭ-'lĭsh-əs). *Highly pleasing or agreeable to the senses of taste and smell.*

Our new, updated definition:
> Delicious (as in *"The Delicious Quick-Trim Diet"*). *Highly pleasing or agreeable to the senses of taste and smell, plus helping you enjoy maximum attractiveness, trimness, vibrant health, and potentially longer life.*

That modern definition of Delicious describes how you've been eating to slim down on D.D., and will continue with variations on D.D. Nutri-Maintenance Eating to attain the thrilling result: *never heavy again.*

Because you have come to prefer the light, naturally superior flavor of good foods, you'll never go back to pre-D.D. fatty, greasy, richly buttered and sauced high-calorie eating. You'll find that you choose D.D. recipes and servings not just because they're low in calories and fat, but because they *taste better*—and because you *feel better*.

Keep in mind always that nutritious, Delicious servings can help keep you looking and feeling your best, enhancing the *total quality* of your life.

MAINTAINING YOUR DESIRED WEIGHT

Here's the day-by-day record, quite typical on D.D., of how an attractive woman aged forty who is five feet three inches tall kept her weight and figure within her height-weight range of 106 to 117 pounds. Her original goal was 110 pounds, down from 135 pounds when she started on her Delicious Diet. She recorded the following steady score week after week:

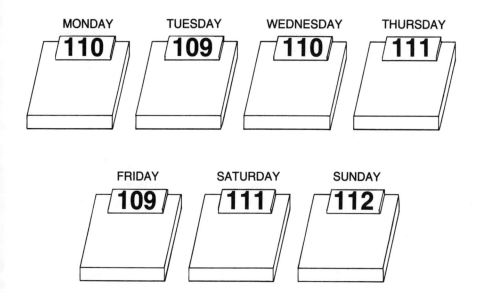

MONDAY 110 TUESDAY 109 WEDNESDAY 110 THURSDAY 111

FRIDAY 109 SATURDAY 111 SUNDAY 112

The fact that her weight varied a pound or two from day to day is not a matter of concern for anyone—as long as you weigh yourself each morning. This woman explained her personal system: she had some weekend dinner dates coming up so she set her eating pattern for the week the following way:

At 110 pounds on Monday, she cut down to prepare for some heavier eating days. She weighed 109 pounds on Tuesday morning, and increased her intake a little. After dining out on Wednesday, she was 111 pounds Thursday morning, so she reduced her intake considerably that day. Company dinners Friday and Saturday brought her up to 112 pounds Sunday morning. She planned to eat less that day, and followed through, so that she'd be back to 110 pounds on Monday morning, thus starting the next week at her desired weight.

In this simple, sensible way she was able to indulge somewhat on social evenings, and still maintain her slim figure. As a result, she kept looking and feeling her best. This is a smart plan that will help you also to stay trim.

"WILL I REGAIN MY EXCESS WEIGHT?"

We can assure you unequivocally that you definitely won't ever be heavy again if you follow the Nutri-Maintenance Guidelines detailed in this book. We have never seen or been able to track down any dependable data supporting statements that "X percentage of people who take off excess weight put it back on again." The percentages given vary dramatically. Unproved statistics and percentages are *un*science that is *non*science that adds up to *nonsense*.

Certainly many people have regained lost weight, but you're not a statistic. You're not a "people." You're an *individual* responsible for your personal weight only. Furthermore, you have something working for you now that was never available before—Delicious Quick-Trim Diets in book form. This can make the enduring difference for you, as for many who have succeeded before by working with the D.D. guidelines.

If you personally, not "people," adhere to D.D. calories-IN-calories-OUT guidelines, you can't help but retain your maximum attractiveness and desired slimness. The proof is not in questionable percentages but in trim, healthy, radiant individuals telling

172

us repeatedly, "I lost my overweight and have stayed trim through your methods"—for up to fifteen years and more.

Repeat, please: "I'm a person, not a percentage. I don't care how many 'percentages' have failed in the past. With D.D., I'll never be heavy again."

EYE ON THE SCALE: FIVE-POUND SWITCH SIGNAL

An essential part of maintaining your desired weight is stepping on an accurate scale every single morning when you wake up— or as often as you can manage that routinely. When you're traveling and staying where a scale isn't in the bathroom, it may be more difficult. One lady who travels a lot weighs herself on the huge freight scales in airports when she lands after an overnight flight (I saw her do this at the airport in Nairobi, Kenya, in East Africa).

Of course you don't have to be that meticulous about a daily weigh-in, but try not to let it lapse too long, either. From now on, *make the scale your sentry*. A dictionary defines sentry as: "A soldier stationed at a place to stand guard and prevent the passage of unauthorized persons." We recommend to you our definition: "The scale is your D.D. sentry stationed to guard your figure and prevent the accumulation of unwanted pounds." If you don't literally watch your weight in actual numbers, those pounds may pile up on you and—*oops!*—you're way overweight again. A psychologist might tell you that you are purposely avoiding the scale because you know that you're eating too much of the wrong high-calorie foods, and don't want the numbers to prove the dire result. For the same reason you may be avoiding the full-length mirror too, even though tight clothes tell you the unhappy truth.

Your good sense affirms that watching for the Five-Pound Switch Signal is an absolute must to keep you trim. When you stop after gaining five pounds, and go right back on your Delicious Diet, you won't put on ten, twenty, or more pounds and uncomfortable inches. But if you don't switch, you'll face the danger of trying to halt a runaway horse—if you don't stop him early, he can go almost beyond control.

Somebody may tell you that a daily weigh-in will make you overly concerned about your weight, and may cause emotional problems (evading the fact that overweight may bring on emotional problems). If that's true for you, we stress again that if you have physical or emotional health problems, you should not be on this or any other diet without your doctor's approval and supervision. Otherwise you certainly can handle and even welcome your morning weigh-in.

As a person in normal health, with pride in your appearance and concern for your maximum well-being, you step on the scale each morning as routinely as brushing your teeth. A digital scale, for one, flashes the numbers to you big and clear—you have the warning and the rest is up to you. If you don't keep those numbers down to where you want them, at least you know the score. How and what you eat that day is your personal responsibility, not the scale's.

If your weight varies a pound or two one way or the other from your desired weight, that's fine, no cause for concern. *But any time your scale registers five pounds more than your desired weight, that's the Five-Pound Switch Signal to switch back to your Delicious Diet until you're down to wanted leanness again.*

Realistically, and knowingly, you'll probably go past the Five-Pound Switch Signal at times when you plan to indulge, as on a vacation. For instance, just before starting to write this book, my wife Natalie and I went off on a fourteen-day cruise, where we ate and drank more than normally.

Upon return, I was nine pounds and she was seven pounds over our desired weights. Immediately we went on the D.D. Three-Day Vegetable Diet, then on the Basic Diet. We were back to desired slimness within a week. We found on Nutri-Maintenance Eating that we appreciated light and flavorful Delicious servings more than ever.

With D.D., you can and will do the same. Eating, vacationing, traveling, are among life's special pleasures. You can enjoy them from now on since you know the way to slim down quickly and deliciously.

It's all-important not to delay returning to your diet at once— *don't wait a single day.* Don't let anything or anybody (including yourself) persuade you to "put it off; a few days won't make any difference." It can make all the difference in growing heavy again, with all the dangerous, unbecoming, unwanted negatives of overweight. Too often despair follows delay.

Here's a typical example of how the D.D. Switch Signal can and will work for you. In this case, a woman of five feet five inches (114 to 125 range) slimmed down on D.D. from 138 pounds to her desired weight of 120 pounds (personal choice). After she attained her wanted weight, here is what happened, as she reported:

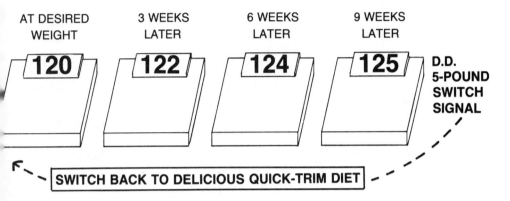

The numbers on the scale show exactly what this smart, motivated woman did, and what many others do as a way of life in order to stay trim. When that Five-Pound Switch Signal flashed the dangerous number "125" on her scale, she went right back on D.D. Within three days she was back to 120 pounds once more. She knew from experience that she could accomplish it on her Delicious Diet. We're certain that she'll stick with her vow, as she has for some time now: *"Never heavy again."*

The signal system couldn't be simpler or clearer for you: Just check the scale—and let the scale check you—day in, day out. Thus, if the numbers warn you through the Five-Pound Switch Signal, starting that day switch back to the Delicious Diet of your choice, step up your daily activity, cut back further on salt, reduce the size of your portions. Perhaps you'll wish to go on the Delicious One-Day Liquid Diet or the Delicious Three-Day Vegetable Diet—your personal decision.

DOWN TO YOUR DESIRED WEIGHT?
OKAY—INDULGE YOURSELF WITHIN REASON

We believe strongly, as you probably do, in the pleasure principle of good living and eating. Yes, enjoying tasty food adds to your gratification, and you should not be deprived. But you know too well that eating rich, fatty, excessively high-calorie foods can be a health disaster, as well as ruining your maximum good looks.

As long as you observe the D.D. Five-Pound Switch Signal, you can certainly enjoy the treats that appeal to you most. You can indulge yourself in "forbidden" dishes and drinks now and then, always within reason, and stay trim as well. The occasional ice cream sundae or Scotch whisky, vodka tonic, or martini will be far more satisfying when you keep your weight down too.

Sylvia and I are living examples of how perfectly the D.D. system can work for anyone. Since I've written a great deal about diet, people who see me enjoying a dish of ice cream tend to ask censoriously, "How can you indulge yourself that way?" I explain (as you can when you're trim), "As long as I'm slim, I eat what I want when I want it. I never stuff myself, hate that overfull feeling. If I gain, I go right back on D.D. low-calorie eating, and I'm soon trim again. The switch system makes it a cinch—it never fails."

Because Sylvia conducts the thriving Creative Food Service, consulting with top food companies, and has written many cookbooks, people ask her, sometimes belligerently, "How can you be so involved with preparing food and yet stay slim?" She says simply, "I not only enjoy delicious food, I respect my health and my appearance. I eat deliciously but never gluttonously. If the scale shows my weight going up, I go into action to take it off immediately." You can do the same, no matter what your situation is.

YOUR GUIDELINES FOR
D.D. NUTRI-MAINTENANCE EATING

Now that you're down to your desired weight, you can eat what you please within specified limitations.

Because you love being trim, you will obey the Five-Pound Switch Signal system, as instructed. Aside from eating and drinking treats that you permit yourself knowingly, here are your general fundamental guidelines for maintaining trimness and maximum good health:

1. *Concentrate on the D.D. lower-calorie foods that you've been eating on your Delicious Quick-Trim Diet*—even though you can now permit yourself some of the higher-calorie items forbidden while you were overweight.

176

No, you don't count calories—that isn't realistic in your demanding daily living. It takes more time, attention, and effort than most individuals are able or willing to apply, and it just doesn't work for most people—so they stay overweight. The simple, practical guidelines here *will* work for you.

You'll find comprehensive calorie tables in Chapter 18 to inform and aid you through ready reference. For instance, if you're not clear about how many calories you'd consume in a serving of asparagus (6 spears, 20 calories) compared with avocado (¼ large size, 90 calories), look them up to decide which to buy when shopping or to order when eating out.

It's always the *total calories daily* that matter in maintaining your trim figure: how many calories IN through eating . . . how many calories OUT due to activity.

If you choose to eat 1,400 total calories a day in ice cream (four ice cream sodas a day as your total calories intake), that contributes no more to your weight than 1,400 calories of chicken, vegetables, and fruits—but of course there's a world of difference in the nutrition you get that day.

The weight/calories chart later in this chapter shows the general balance with respect to weight, height, and calories. Coupled with the D.D. Guidelines, and the detailed data in Chapter 18, you have all the information required to help keep you trim.

2. *Remember always that fat is your enemy.* The only fat the normal adult body needs is a small amount of linoleic acid. It's contained naturally in a number of foods on D.D., including chicken, turkey, fish, shellfish, meat, cottage cheese, eggs, whole-wheat and whole-grain breads, and nuts. So there's little concern ever about whether your body is being fed enough fat. The main problem is too much fat.

One precaution you should keep observing when you eat is to trim any visible fat and skin off poultry, fish (some have fatty skin), and meats; you'll still be getting more than enough "invisible" fat from many foods.

3. *Stay away from quantities of greasy foods* such as deep-fried chicken, shrimp, potatoes, and other fried foods (aside from treats you select such as occasional French fries with a hamburger, as discussed later). When trim, you can permit yourself limited amounts of butter, margarine, and vegetable oil—but don't go overboard lest you become overweight and less healthy again.

Take a tip from athlete Satchel Paige, noted for his phenomenal stamina as a fifty-nine-year-old major-league pitcher. He advised, "Avoid fried meats, which angry up the blood." By using reasonable restraint and good sense, you won't "angry up your blood" with excess fat intake that puts on excess pounds in a hurry.

4. *Beware of loading on rich additives*—high-calorie mayonnaise and other dressings, gravies, sauces. Make it a habit to use dressings "on the side," so you get the taste you want without submerging the fine natural flavor. If you're going to bury the inherent taste of good foods, you might as well be heaping fattening dressings on torn-up scraps of paper towels as far as total flavor is concerned.

5. *Never overuse salt and sugar.* With certain medical conditions, salt and sugar act as poisons—and too much may be harmful to most people. Avoid highly-salted, salt-cured, salt-pickled, and smoked foods. Consider salt and sugar substitutes, never going overboard on those either. Fortunately, there now are many low-sodium or no-sodium items, and sugar-free or no-sugar-added foods available. Look for them and read labels carefully for sugar and salt contents.

6. *Apply caution with desserts, too.* There's no reason why you can't enjoy treats once you're trim—but do it the way slim, discriminating gourmets do: take a smaller amount and savor every nibble, each morsel. Enjoy it s-l-o-w-l-y—no more gobble and gulp and it's gone! A slim slice of yummy homemade pie appreciated slowly bit by bit can be much more satisfying than a thick slice of the same pie crammed in heedlessly.

An ounce of discretion is worth far more than the excess pounds. Is a heavily buttered sweet roll really worth a bloated, bulging belly to you? *Apply the tradeoff system.* If you have the buttered sweet roll, which totals about 200 calories, skip another food that would add about the same number of calories that day—such as a hamburger, bowl of pea soup, a couple of beers; check the calories chart in Chapter 18, if you like.

7. *Sip a glass of wine or hard spirits* if you enjoy them—but again it's the better part of taste enjoyment to sip slowly. When you gulp, the flavor passes by before you're even aware of it. Moderation in drinking is far healthier—and no high-proof headaches or potential liver damage. Consider switching to the new, lighter wines, liquors, and beers—considerably lower in calories, and found satisfying by many people.

It's always up to you to decide how to use your daily calorie quotient. You could have a three-ounce glass of "light" dry wine at about 50 calories (7 percent alcohol), a regular dry wine at about 75 calories (9.4 percent alcohol) or sweet wine at about 120 calories (9.4 percent alcohol).

Comparably, distilled spirits run about 70 calories per ounce for 80 proof, up to 85 calories for 100 proof. A liqueur such as apricot brandy is 90 to 100 calories per ounce. It's your choice, based primarily on your taste preferences—and the score on your scale each morning.

8. *Check the size of your portions.* Don't let yourself or a hostess heap your plate with oversize servings. Most of us have the urge to "clean off the plate" rather than leave some food. It's more effective maintenance eating to start with less, then go back for more if wanted; usually you can be satisfied without taking more.

In restaurants, there's great overweight-again danger in ordering from the full-course menu instead of choosing from á la carte listings. By resisting the lure of getting more food and saving what amounts to pennies, you help save yourself from adding excess pounds.

9. *Be careful about snacks and other extras* where the calories add up—a grab here, a gobble there. Often you consume handy nibbles without realizing how many fattening calories you're cramming in—and without really enjoying the extras. Be aware—and employ the swap system, avoiding additional ounces.

For example, you can enjoy some of the tasty breads and rolls on Nutri-Maintenance Eating by substituting them for other servings. Beware particularly in restaurants where, unless you're alert, you may find yourself reaching into the bread basket and loading in the calories as you chat while awaiting your order. A couple of rolls and butter can total 300 calories or more—all settling on your waistline and hips sooner or later. Inflation indeed—but this time it's self-controllable.

Further food for thought: A breadstick adds about 30 calories, and a slice of Italian bread, very tasty, is about 85 calories—but if you load it with butter or margarine you not only subdue the inherent flavor of the bread itself, you also push the total calorie count for that one buttered slice up to about 120 calories.

It's easy to figure out how the selection system can serve you well. In that same restaurant you might prefer to have a cup of consommé, about 25 calories, and a slice of garlic bread of 120 calories—both for a lesser calorie total than a bowl of thick minestrone soup of 250 to 300 calories.

So watch carefully what you eat, for your health and waistline's sake. Be attentive every day, one day at a time, monitoring yourself against indiscreet choosing of servings and snacks. Keep reminding yourself that *overweight can "snack" up on you.*

10. *Never overload your stomach or eat one bite more beyond satisfying your appetite.* Nobody but you can know when you reach that point of feeling reasonably full without feeling stuffed. Keep in mind the example of a beautiful friend of ours, an important scientist, who enjoys a taste of a rich dessert, then puts down her spoon with finality and says, "The calories just aren't worth ruining my looks and health."

Ask yourself before you reach out for more: "Do I value a fudge brownie more than my figure?" You're likely to find yourself stopping time after time and saying happily, *"The calories aren't worth it."*

And when you reach out with a serving spoon, don't lie to yourself about the size of portions. You know the difference between "small," "medium," and "large" portions. You may minimize the size of a serving and the calorie total, but your stomach and your scale won't be fooled.

11. *Benefit from D.D. low-calorie servings for the rest of your life—* just as you've enjoyed them on your Delicious Diet. D.D. recipes will be a constant asset in maintaining your weight, too. As you know now, D.D. dishes are loaded with flavor but not with excess calories.

Other tips for keeping trim and fit: Drink lots of water daily. Fill and refresh yourself with sugar-free carbonated beverages, decaffeinated (and some regular) coffee and the great variety of teas; low-sodium, low-calorie broths; low-sodium, low-calorie vegetable and tomato juices.

Don't forget the many raw vegetables, low in calories but high in nutrition and satisfying to your appetite. You know from experience through your weight-loss period that they can be especially delicious and satisfyingly enhanced with flavorful, low-calorie D.D. dips.

A sugar-free gelatin dessert at only 10 calories a portion can be a filling, gratifying snack, particularly when prepared the D.D. ways.

Scan the food pages and shop for new calorie-reduced items, increasingly available at supermarkets and other stores. But always make sure to note the number of calories per serving in the small type on the package; that's very important, because words like "Lower in Calories" in large type on the label may not be borne out by the actual small-size *numbers* in type.

HOW MANY CALORIES TO
MAINTAIN YOUR DESIRED WEIGHT?

You didn't count calories on your Delicious Quick-Trim Diet, nor is it necessary that you count calories on D.D. Nutri-Maintenance Eating. That's the case even though calories do count.

However, if you are fascinated by the details and mathematics of counting calories, do so by all means. Realize nevertheless that your morning weigh-in on the scale reveals your precise poundage at that moment, as calorie counts cannot do.

To help you assess and compare calories in foodstuffs and liquids, you'll find an extensive, sufficiently complete checklist of calories, protein, fat, and carbohydrates in Chapter 18. Comprehensive for everyday eating purposes, it contains some 600 listings of foods and liquids.

Just by comparing the items and their calorie, fat, and other listed counts can be a considerable help in keeping your weight under control through D.D. Nutri-Maintenance Eating. Look it over now for a moment if you wish, and note instantly how you can manage your total daily calorie intake readily through comparing and selecting.

You'll see that you don't have to reduce the *amount* of the food you eat—as long as you choose the lower-calorie items in each category. The following examples show how *lower-calorie selectivity* can work for you:

MAIN COURSE *(4 oz.): chicken, 200 cal.—turkey, 230 cal.—striped bass, 120 cal.—shrimp, 100 cal.—tuna (canned in water), 150 cal.—salmon (canned, drained), 180 cal.—beef steak (lean), 250 cal.—lamb (lean), 210 cal.—veal (lean), 240 cal.*
FRUITS: *apple (medium), 70 cal.—banana (medium), 100 cal.— cantaloupe, 40 cal.—grapefruit half, 50 cal.—orange (medium), 60 cal.*

VEGETABLES: *asparagus, 6 spears, 20 cal.—avocado half (large), 180 cal.—1 cup broccoli, 50 cal.—1 cup carrots, 20 cal.—1 head lettuce, 30–70 cal.—potato (medium), 100 cal.—1 cup spinach, 45*

181

cal.—sweet potato (medium), 160 cal.—tomato (medium), 30 cal.—
1 cup watercress, 10 cal.
MILK *(1 cup): buttermilk, 99 cal.—skim milk, 86 cal.—skim, 1 %*
fat, 102 cal.—whole milk, 157 cal. (note that a cup of nutritious
skim milk is 70 calories less than whole milk)

GRAIN PRODUCTS *(½ cup): farina, 55 cal.—oatmeal, 75 cal.—corn*
flakes, 50 cal.—wheat flakes, 45 cal.—sugared cereals, about 75–
100 cal.—granolas, about 200–250 cal.—macaroni, rice, spaghetti,
about 100 cal.—bread (slice), about 60 cal.—Melba toast (slice), 15
cal.

These items are a start for you. Use the numbers as a general
gauge rather than exact counts. Obviously, one four-ounce lean
steak might be more or fewer calories than another four-ounce
cut of lean steak—but the small difference isn't significant with
respect to your weight.

Decide according to your own preferences how desserts, pas-
tries, candies, and other sweets fit your eating pattern in order
to stay within your daily calorie allowance. If you like wines and
spirits, you have a wide choice in calorie range in wines, whiskies,
vodka, gin, cocktails, brandies, liqueurs; beers can vary from under
100 calories per 12-ounce glass of "light" beer to 150 to 200 calories
per 12-ounce glass for regular and imported beers.

It couldn't be simpler: You can make your personal choices of
what to eat and drink each day, and still maintain your desired
weight. All you have to do is step on your scale first thing each
morning. The numbers there tell you whether to cut down on
calories or allow yourself a little more leeway.

Now you know—the rest is up to you. If you don't keep that
daily check on the scale—and obey the D.D. Five-Pound Switch
Signal—you may pass a full-length mirror someday soon, glance
at the person there, and scream, "Help, a fat woman (man) has
taken over my body!"

The figures here provide the range of calories on which most
people maintain weight according to height. These numbers are
for your general understanding and guidance—along with useful
information on protein, fat, and carbohydrate content.

If, according to the chart, your daily total consumption of
calories is far above the top range for your height, you will undoubtedly put on excess weight and ungainly bulk. Unhappily,

D.D. ADULT WEIGHT CHART AND MATCHING CALORIES
. . . Desirable Weight (Completely Unclothed) . . .

	WOMEN			MEN	
Daily Calories	Range in Pounds		Height	Range in Pounds	Daily Calories
1,030–1,130	86 . . . 94		4'8"	94 . . . 100	1,220–1,300
1,070–1,170	89 . . . 96		4'9"	96 . . . 103	1,250–1,340
1,100–1,200	91 . . . 98		4'10"	97 . . . 105	1,260–1,370
1,140–1,250	94 . . . 102		4'11"	100 . . . 108	1,300–1,400
1,170–1,280	96 . . . 104		5'	102 . . . 112	1,330–1,460
1,200–1,320	98 . . . 107		5'1"	105 . . . 118	1,370–1,540
1,210–1,350	100 . . . 110		5'2"	110 . . . 124	1,430–1,610
1,270–1,400	106 . . . 117		5'3"	115 . . . 130	1,500–1,690
1,330–1,470	111 . . . 122		5'4"	120 . . . 135	1,560–1,760
1,370–1,500	114 . . . 125		5'5"	125 . . . 140	1,630–1,820
1,420–1,560	118 . . . 130		5'6"	130 . . . 145	1,690–1,890
1,440–1,620	120 . . . 135		5'7"	135 . . . 150	1,760–1,950
1,520–1,680	126 . . . 140		5'8"	140 . . . 155	1,820–2,020
1,560–1,740	130 . . . 145		5'9"	145 . . . 160	1,890–2,080
1,620–1,780	135 . . . 148		5'10"	150 . . . 165	1,950–2,150
1,680–1,860	140 . . . 155		5'11"	155 . . . 170	2,020–2,210
1,740–1,920	145 . . . 160		6'	160 . . . 175	2,080–2,280
1,800–1,980	150 . . . 165		6'1"	165 . . . 180	2,150–2,340
1,860–2,020	155 . . . 168		6'2"	170 . . . 185	2,210–2,410
1,920–2,070	160 . . . 172		6'3"	175 . . . 190	2,280–2,470
1,980–2,140	165 . . . 178		6'4"	180 . . . 195	2,340–2,540
2,040–2,200	170 . . . 183		6'5"	185 . . . 200	2,410–2,600
2,100–2,260	175 . . . 188		6'6"	190 . . . 205	2,470–2,670
2,160–2,300	180 . . . 192		6'7"	195 . . . 210	2,540–2,740
2,220–2,350	185 . . . 196		6'8"	200 . . . 215	2,600–2,800

you will quite definitely stay overweight, becoming heavier and increasing the hazards to your health, unless you take off the excess pounds in a hurry. You should take action immediately: Go right back on one of the Delicious Diets. Then adhere closely to Nutri-Maintenance Guidelines, a sure formula for staying trim.

For the sake of your figure and good health, note the weight range for your height, then select your target number and maintain it lifelong.

THE INFLUENCE OF ACTIVITY

How active you are—that is, how many energy calories you expend in walking, jogging, exercising, work, or other activities—influences your weight, since all movement (even the act of breathing) uses up some calories. You'd need a computer to keep an accurate account of the calories taken in through eating and the calories used up through activity. You still wouldn't have a predictably exact weight result because individual variations in body functioning influence weight loss and gain.

Your only real authority and guide for your daily precise weight is an accurate scale.

TYPICAL DAY OF D.D. NUTRI-MAINTENANCE EATING

Here's an example of how you'll maintain your desired weight through D.D. Nutri-Maintenance Eating. You don't count calories. The following listing shows just about how much you can eat and still stay slim—the calories are shown simply to indicate how specific foods apply to the daily total that keeps you trim.

As you'll note in this typical Nutri-Maintenance day, you may use D.D. recipes if you or someone in your household likes to cook, or you may prepare whatever other dishes you prefer, following D.D. Guidelines.

In this case, the person exemplified is a woman 5 feet 4 inches tall. She reduced to her desired weight of 120 pounds (from 137 pounds), which she can maintain generally on about 1,400 calories. Here's her eating on a typical day:

Breakfast

	calories
Half cantaloupe	40
½ cup plain low-fat yogurt	60
½ cup blueberries (mixed in the yogurt)	45
Coffee (dash of skim milk, artificial sweetener)	10
	155

Midmorning Snack

Pound cake, slice	130
Tea with lemon	0
	130

Lunch

*D.D. Tuna-Mushroom Salad	220
*D.D. Fresh Fruit Cup	120
No-sugar, no-caffeine cola (or other flavor) soda	5
	345

184

Dinner

Chilled dry white wine	75
*D.D. Vegetable Broth	10
*D.D. Rock Cornish Hen à L'Orange	256
*D.D. Green Beans with Celery	30
*D.D. Chocolate-Chunk Mousse	120
Tea with lemon	0
	491

The total day's eating here amounts to 1,121 calories. This leaves a "deficit" of about 300 calories, which you might think of as "special treat calories" for indulging yourself with food that was forbidden while you were on the Quick-Loss dieting. Of course you need not eat anything extra, thus allowing yourself the option of going over your daily 1,400 calories total the next day (perhaps a Saturday when you'd be dining out).

Or, you might like to have a baked apple in the evening (70 calories), some Camembert cheese and crackers (130 calories), an extra-dry martini (100 calories), and a few assorted hors d'oeuvres, (100 calories).

A further variation might be treating yourself during the day to an ice cream sundae (200 calories) or, if you enjoy vegetables and fruits, you can use the 200 calories for added vegetables at lunch and dinner or for munching fruit at or between meals.

It should be clear to you now that on D.D. Nutri-Maintenance Eating, your daily choices are your own. Always keep in mind these fundamental guidelines for sustaining your beautifully slimmed figure:

- *Fat* is your enemy; keep it to a minimum.
- Use only limited amounts of *high-calorie additives*—butter, margarine, oils, and so on.
- Avoid *greasy foods*; restrict yourself to small servings, if any.
- Don't load up on *rich dressings, gravies,* and *sauces.*
- Never overuse *sugars* and *salt.*
- Restrain intake of *desserts* and high-calorie *sweet drinks.*
- Limit your use of *alcoholic drinks.*
- Benefit from Delicious, nutritious D.D. *recipes* and available *low-calorie foods.* (If you're doubtful about whether a food is high or low in calories, look it up in Chapter 18—or on the package.)
- *Never overload your stomach . . . instant danger!*
- Plan and engage in *daily continuous-action exercise* (15 minutes or more of sustained movement such as brisk walking or

physical work) to the extent of your ability, *but never over-extend yourself.*

CONSTANTLY REMIND YOURSELF: THE SCALE AND D.D. FIVE-POUND SWITCH SIGNAL ARE YOUR DAILY WATCHDOGS AND FRIENDS

Because you are not a robot, we must emphasize again that your body has no built-in calorie-counting computer. One and one doesn't always add up to two in the human system.

Therefore, even counting calories cannot assure that you'll stay trim. The one positive number you can count on is the one that you register on your accurate weight scale. Make your scale check-in as much a morning habit as brushing your teeth—and take the advised D.D. action accordingly each day.

D.D. NUTRI-MAINTENANCE RECIPES

This is not a cookbook, it's planned specifically in every word to: (1) reduce you swiftly and healthfully with effective Delicious Quick-Trim Diets; (2) keep you trim "forever" through Nutri-Maintenance Eating as detailed in this chapter.

Always be guarded—read recipes cautiously in any cookbook, magazine, newspaper, and so on. Many recipes go overboard on calories, thereby promoting *overweight* through excessive calorie content. Examine even so-called low-calorie recipes carefully for total calories. As D.D. recipes in this book prove conclusively, great taste need not mean overloading with high-calorie ingredients.

Scanning just one well-known cookbook of "family recipes" reveals many that include large quantities of ingredients like the following, frighteningly high in calories—but, of course, they don't list enormous calorie totals:

	calories
1½ cups mayonnaise	2,400
1 cup butter or margarine	1,800
1 cup vegetable oil	2,000
2 cups sugar	1,540
1½ cups heavy cream	1,200

186

To repeat, don't take it for granted that a recipe is truly low in calories just because it has a name like "Reducing Diet Recipe." As an example, this listing appeared on a newspaper food page as "Diet Recipe for Roquefort Salad Dressing . . . using butter-milk cuts calories." But here's how the recipe added up in total calories (which were not shown anywhere):

	calories
¼ cup firmly packed Roquefort cheese	230
¼ cup mayonnaise	450
½ cup buttermilk	45
½ teaspoon paprika; pepper and salt to taste	0

Being knowledgeable and careful, you'd realize now that sub-stituting buttermilk for whole milk saves only 45 calories. The significant total for the so-called Reducing Diet Recipe is 725 ca-lories, *over 45 calories per tablespoon*. In contrast, D.D. salad dress-ings, which are delicious, are *as low as 5 calories per tablespoon*. It pays in fewer pounds and inches, and in smaller clothing sizes, always to check and compare.

The D.D. Nutri-Maintenance recipes that follow allow the kinds of servings that enable you to indulge deliciously but sen-sibly once you're trim. They will satisfy your need for variety yet help you keep at your desired weight. D.D. recipes cut calories up to half and more, without cutting satisfying taste.

Keep the difference in mind: The Delicious Quick-Trim Diets cut your intake down to about 1,000 calories daily in order to take off your excess pounds swiftly. Now that you are trim, you can take in more calories with dishes such as these sample D.D. Nutri-Maintenance recipes—and still stay slim.

Summing up: All the recipes anywhere in this book, including those for Delicious dieting in Chapter 12, are delectable and nu-tritious for Nutri-Maintenance Eating as well. Such servings elim-inate extra unneeded, unwanted calories while enhancing the fine natural flavors in foods. They help make the crucial difference for you between a bulky, bloated, overweight body—and a trim, attractive figure.

TO PREPARE OR NOT TO PREPARE

If you make the D.D. Key Recipes such as *D.D. "Mayo," *D.D. Vegetable Broth, *D.D. "Crème Fraîche," or *D.D. Salad Dressing, you know how much they add to meals, and to simplifying the preparation of many other recipes. However, if you are not a cook-ahead type, substitute a purchased product—low-calorie mayonnaise, or low-sodium, low-fat broth, or yogurt or other alternates indicated in the individual recipes. Once you get into the swing of D.D. low-calorie, low-fat, lower-sodium cooking, you will want to make this your permanent cookstyle.

D.D. NUTRI-MAINTENANCE RECIPES

D.D. CHOCOLATE-CHUNK MOUSSE

This delectable dessert was preferred in a small group-taste comparison over a rich, creamy chocolate mousse totaling 400 calories for the same size serving, prepared from a recipe in a famous French chef's cookbook. Try this D.D. version as an example of how you can cut calories per serving to one-quarter the calories for the same type of dish, enjoy it more, and yet keep slim and feel wonderful about staying at your desired weight.

5 ounces semisweet chocolate
6 egg whites
Pinch salt
2 egg yolks

2 tablespoons almond, cherry, or
orange liqueur
Strawberries or thin orange slices
for garnish

Melt 4 ounces of the chocolate until limp but not runny. Cut remaining 1 ounce of chocolate into very small chunks. Beat whites very stiff with a pinch of salt. With same beater, beat yolks with liqueur, beating very thoroughly until yolks are thick, pale, and fluffy. Add yolk mixture to chocolate and stir together. Fold in chocolate chunks. Fold in beaten egg whites lightly but thoroughly. Chill 3 hours. Serve garnished with strawberries or thin orange slices. *Makes 8 servings, 120 calories per serving.*

D.D. FUDGY CHOCOLATE MERINGUES

4 egg whites, at room temperature
1 teaspoon vanilla
⅛ teaspoon cream of tartar
  or ½ teaspoon white vinegar

Pinch salt
¾ cup granulated sugar
½ cup unsweetened cocoa powder

Beat egg whites with vanilla, cream of tartar or vinegar, and salt until soft peaks form. Beat in sugar 1 tablespoon at a time, reserving 2 tablespoons. Continue to beat until meringue is stiff and shiny. Combine the reserved 2 tablespoons sugar with cocoa in a sifter and sift on top of meringue. Carefully fold in cocoa mixture.

Drop by tablespoonfuls (or use pastry bag and star tube) onto a baking sheet that has been lined with foil or baking parchment. Bake in a 200° F (or less) oven about 1½ hours, or until meringues are firm and lift easily from foil. Remove from oven and cool on baking sheet. Store lightly covered in a dry place. *Makes 40 meringues, 30 calories each.*

D.D. APRICOT MOUSSE

8 ounces dried apricots
5 egg whites
1 tablespoon almond liqueur

10 tablespoons *D.D. Ricotta or
  Cottage Crème

Place apricots in small saucepan with water to cover. Stew until the fruit is tender. Cool in liquid. Place apricots and their liquid in food processor or blender container. Blend until smooth. Turn into a large bowl. Beat egg whites until stiff, then beat in almond liqueur. Fold about one fourth of egg whites thoroughly into the apricot puree; fold remaining egg whites in lightly. Pour into serving dish or individual dessert glasses. Garnish with ricotta or cottage crème—1 tablespoon per serving. *makes 10 servings, 83 calories per serving.*

D.D. SKINNY APPLE TART

1¼ cups flour
½ tablespoon active dry yeast
½ cup very warm water
1 teaspoon sugar or honey
2 tablespoons sweet butter

3 Golden Delicious apples, cored,
   peeled, and sliced very thin
   (food processor excels)
3 tablespoons apricot preserves
2 tablespoons water

Sift flour onto square of waxed paper. Combine yeast, warm water, and honey in bowl of food processor, or in mixing bowl. Add about a third of the flour and whirl briefly. Let stand 10 minutes, or until bubbly. Add remaining flour and butter and whirl about 30 seconds to combine. Dough should form a ball that cleans side of bowl. Remove dough, place on lightly floured board, and shape into a smooth ball. Pat into flat round, then roll into an oval shape about 10 by 15 inches, pulling into shape. Roll up on pin, place on cookie sheet, and tuck edge of dough under to form rounded lip. Let stand in warm place to rise slightly while you prepare the filling.

Arrange apple slices in a neat pattern over crust in thin, overlapping slices. Combine apricot preserves with 2 tablespoons water, bring to a boil, and spoon over apple slices. Bake at 400° F until glazed and golden, about 20 minutes. *Makes 12 servings, 98 calories per serving.*

D.D. APPLE STRUDEL

4 apples (Granny Smith or Rome
   Beauty), peeled and cored, cut
   into small cubes
Juice of ½ lemon
2 sheets phyllo or strudel dough
   (available in packages, generally
   refrigerated)

2 tablespoons melted butter
4 tablespoons stale bread crumbs
2 tablespoons raisins
2 tablespoons granulated sugar
½ teaspoon ground cinnamon

(cont.)

Prepare apple cubes and drop into lemon juice combined with cold water to cover. Unfold one sheet of phyllo dough on moistened towel, placed lengthwise away from you. Brush with 1 tablespoon butter. Sprinkle with 2 tablespoons of bread crumbs. Place second sheet over first, repeating spreading as above. Drain apple cubes. Add raisins and most of sugar and cinnamon. Toss all to combine, then heap along edge of dough closest to you. Roll up like a jelly roll, lifting the towel to help dough roll. Roll onto cookie sheet, brush top with remaining butter, and sprinkle with remaining sugar and cinnamon. Bake at 400° F about 25 minutes, until golden brown. *Makes 10 servings at 78 calories per serving or 8 servings at 98 calories per serving.*

NOTE: Since some dough packages hold four leaves, it is tempting to make two strudels, and freeze one for later use—the next time you plan a dinner party!

D.D. PLUM CLAFOUTI
(French-Style Cobbler)

½ cup flour
1 tablespoon honey
2 eggs
½ teaspoon double-acting baking
  powder
1 cup skim milk
¼ teaspoon salt

2 tablespoons *D.D. "Crème
  Fraîche" or plain low-fat yogurt
2 cups halved and seeded small
  fresh purple or red plums
2 tablespoons plum or other
  brandy

In a large mixing bowl, combine flour, honey, eggs, baking powder, skim milk, salt, and "crème fraîche." Pour into shallow 9-inch casserole or ovenproof skillet sprayed with vegetable cooking spray. Bake about 5 minutes at 350° F, to set bottom slightly. Arrange plums on top, sprinkle with brandy, return to oven, and bake about 30 minutes longer, until set and golden brown. Serve warm or cold. *Makes 8 servings, 105 calories per serving.*

D.D. YOGURT CHEESE PIE

Crust:
8 *light rye wafers*
2 *tablespoons (packed) brown*
  sugar

Dash salt
2 *teaspoons melted butter*
1 *teaspoon water*

Filling:
1 *envelope (1 tablespoon)*
  unflavored gelatin
3 *tablespoons granulated sugar*
⅛ *teaspoon salt*
¼ *cup water*
½ *teaspoon grated lemon rind*

2 *tablespoons lemon juice*
¾ *cup plain low-fat yogurt*
1 *cup low-fat ricotta or cottage*
  cheese, sieved
1 *egg white*

For the crust, press the wafers between 2 sheets of waxed paper with a rolling pin to make crumbs, or whirl them in a blender or food processor. Add remaining ingredients for crust and blend well. Press mixture onto bottom and sides of an 8-inch pie pan. Bake for 8 minutes at 375° F. Cool before filling.

For the filling, mix gelatin, sugar, and salt in small pan. Add water and stir over low heat until clear. Remove mixture from heat. In blender container or food processor, combine gelatin mixture with grated lemon rind, lemon juice, yogurt, and ricotta or cottage cheese. Whirl smooth (or beat all together with rotary beater). Chill until the mixture begins to thicken. Beat the egg white until stiff, and fold in. Pour into the rye crumb crust and place in refrigerator to set for several hours before serving. *Makes 8 servings, 98 calories per serving.*

D.D. SEAFOOD SEVICHE

1 pound bay scallops or fish fillets
   cut into ½ inch pieces (bass or
   porgy or even whiting do fine)
¾ cup lime or lemon juice
2 large tomatoes, peeled and
   chopped
1 onion, finely chopped

1 small fresh hot red or green
   pepper, seeded and finely
   chopped
1 teaspoon chopped mint leaves or
   parsley
Salt, pepper (optional)

Put the scallops or fish pieces into a glass or china bowl. Pour lime or lemon juice over, cover, and refrigerate overnight. Drain the fish, reserving the juice. In the bowl, combine the fish with tomatoes, onion, hot pepper, mint leaves or parsley, and ¼ cup of the reserved juice. Season to taste with salt and pepper. Serve in a bowl lined with lettuce leaves or in small shells. *Makes 4 main dish servings at 67 calories per serving, or 8 hors d'oeuvre servings at 34 calories per serving.*

D.D. SHRIMP SALAD

½ pound small shrimp
1 scallion, sliced, or 1 onion slice
1 tablespoon soy sauce
½ cup water
¼ cup *D.D. "Mayo"
¼ cup seeded and diced fresh ripe
   plum tomatoes

½ cup canned water chestnuts,
   drained and sliced
1 tablespoon chopped chives or
   scallion top
½ teaspoon grated fresh ginger
Watercress

Clean raw shrimp, reserving shells. Cook shells with scallion and soy sauce in ½ cup water, about 5 minutes. Strain liquid over shrimp in pan and simmer 3 to 4 minutes, just until shrimp turn

(cont.)

opaque and pink. Cool shrimp in liquid. Add 2 tablespoons of cooking liquid to "mayo." Add tomatoes to shrimp, along with water chestnuts and chives. Add ginger to mayo mixture, and combine lightly with shrimp and vegetables. Chill and serve with watercress. *Makes 4 appetizer servings at 81 calories each or 2 main servings at 163 calories each.*

D.D. GUACAMOLE

Serve this as a dip for oven-warmed tortilla pieces . . . and stop after a few dips. In Mexico, guacamole is called "poor man's butter." It is high in fat—but lower in calories than butter!

1 ripe avocado
Juice of 1 small lime
2 shallots, chopped
1 small tomato, peeled, seeded,
    and chopped

½ fresh hot red pepper, chopped
3 to 4 sprays chopped fresh
    coriander or parsley

Mash avocado coarsely with fork, mashing in lime juice. Combine with chopped shallots, tomato, hot pepper, and coriander or parsley. *Makes 1⅓ cups, 20 calories per tablespoon.*

D.D. SKINNY MUSHROOM QUICHE

4 sheets of phyllo or strudel dough
2 thin slices prosciutto ham
2 medium onions, diced
½ pound mushrooms, sliced
2 tablespoons *D.D. Chicken
    Broth or nonfat low-sodium
    chicken broth
2 egg whites

2 eggs
1 cup *D.D. Ricotta or Cottage
    Crème
1 cup skim milk
1 teaspoon curry powder
Salt and freshly ground white
    pepper
½ cup grated Swiss cheese

(cont.)

Layer 4 dough leaves on a nonstick cookie pan or jelly-roll pan (14 x 10 inches). Fold edges under to make a smooth rim around the pan. Cover the phyllo with a damp towel to prevent drying. Trim fat from ham and dice meat, then scatter over pastry. Wilt diced onion in small pan with 1 tablespoon of the hot broth, and scatter over ham. Cook mushrooms in remaining 1 tablespoon broth until browned, and scatter over onion. Beat egg whites until foamy. Add to them the whole eggs, ricotta or cottage crème, skim milk, and seasonings to taste and beat to combine. Pour custard into pastry shell. Sprinkle with cheese. Bake in hot oven (425° F) until pastry is golden and custard is set. Cut into rectangles, about 3 x 1½ inches. *Makes 27 hors d'oeuvre servings, 34 calories per serving.*

D.D. EGGPLANT PARMESAN

*1¼ cups *D.D. Tomato Sauce*
1 eggplant (1¼ pound)
1 tablespoon vegetable oil

¼ cup grated Parmesan cheese
¼ pound low-fat mozzarella cheese
(or part feta cheese), grated

Prepare tomato sauce or puree canned plum tomatoes with basil and onion to taste. Wash eggplant and cut off stem end. Slice unpeeled eggplant ½ inch thick. Place on oiled 13½ x 11½-inch baking sheet. Turn oiled sides up and bake in 400° F oven about 20 minutes, until slices are tender when pierced with a fork. Spread ¼ cup of tomato sauce in 9 x 6-inch baking dish. Add layer of half the eggplant slices. Spoon remaining tomato sauce over, sprinkle with grated Parmesan cheese. Add remaining eggplant slices and tomato sauce. Top with grated mozzarella cheese. Bake at 375° F for 20 minutes, until bubbling and cheese is melted. *Makes 4 servings, about 200 calories per serving.*

Microwave Directions: Spread oil in 13 x 9 x 2-inch glass baking dish. Turn eggplant slices to coat, then cover with waxed paper. Cook on high about 5 minutes, turn to cook 4 minutes longer, or until slices are tender. Assemble in microwave baking dish as directed above. Cook, uncovered, 10 minutes.

D.D. GARDEN VEGGIE SLAW

2 cups coarsely shredded low-
  calorie raw vegetables (Use any
  combination of zucchini,
  cauliflower, green beans,
  broccoli, yellow squash,
  radishes, green pepper, green
  onion, celery)
1 cup each red and green cabbage
2 tablespoons white or wine
  vinegar

¼ cup *D.D. Vegetable Broth or
  nonfat broth or plain or low-fat
  yogurt
1 tablespoon prepared mustard
¼ teaspoon freshly ground pepper
2 tablespoons *D.D. "Mayo"
½ teaspoon caraway seeds
  (optional)

Toss shredded vegetables in large bowl to combine. In a separate bowl place vinegar, broth, mustard, pepper, and "mayo"; blend with fork or wire whisk. Pour over vegetables. Sprinkle caraway seeds over all and stir with fork to coat. Refrigerate until serving time. *Makes 8 servings, 27 calories per serving.*

D.D. TURKEY STEAKS FORESTIÈRE

1 pound boneless turkey breast
  meat
1 tablespoon chopped shallots or
  Spanish onion
1 tablespoon butter or vegetable oil

½ cup sliced mushrooms
½ cup *D.D. Tomato Sauce
Juice of ½ lemon
¼ cup dry white wine

Buy whole turkey breast meat fresh or frozen for this dish. Trim the skin and any sinews from breast meat (reserve them for use in stock). It will be easier to accomplish next step, cutting meat into thin slices, if you chill turkey first, about 15 minutes in the freezer. Cut frozen meat into thin diagonal slices across the grain.

Cook the shallots or onion in butter or oil over moderate heat, stirring until they are glazed. Add mushrooms and cook until golden. Remove vegetables from pan. Sear the turkey meat quickly on both

(cont.)

sides in the seasoned butter. Add tomato sauce, lemon juice, wine, and glazed vegetables. Reduce and simmer about 10 minutes, until the turkey steaks are cooked through. Serve with ½ cup green spinach noodles per portion. *Makes 4 servings, 189 calories per serving.*

D.D. SUKIYAKI

½ pound round steak
1 small onion
2 stalks celery
¼ pound mushrooms
3 scallions
½ red bell pepper
½ can (¼ cup) water chestnuts, drained

2 teaspoons vegetable oil
¼ cup *D.D. Vegetable Broth or nonfat low-sodium vegetable broth
½ teaspoon grated fresh ginger or ¼ teaspoon ground ginger
2 tablespoons soy sauce
¼ pound fresh spinach leaves

Chill steak briefly in freezer. Cut into very thin diagonal slices across the grain. Cut onion, celery, mushrooms, scallions, red pepper, and water chestnuts into thin diagonal slices or strips. Heat the oil in a large skillet or wok. Brown the meat slices quickly, then push to one side. Add onion, celery, mushrooms, scallions, and red pepper. Cook 3 minutes, stir-tossing. Add water chestnuts, broth, ginger, and soy sauce; add spinach leaves. Cover and cook 2 minutes. *Makes 3 servings, 187 calories per serving.*

D.D. LOW-CALORIE SPINACH SOUFFLÉ

1 package (10 ounces) frozen
  spinach, partially thawed
2 tablespoons chopped onion
½ cup sliced mushrooms
2 tablespoons low-fat cottage
  cheese
2 tablespoons grated Parmesan
  cheese

⅛ teaspoon freshly ground nutmeg
2 egg yolks
5 egg whites
2 tablespoons lemon juice
3 tablespoons *D.D. Tomato
  Sauce or plum tomatoes pureed
  with basil and onion to taste

Press spinach through sieve to remove excess liquid. Place in food processor or mixing bowl. Add onion, mushrooms, cottage cheese, and 1 tablespoon of the Parmesan cheese. Whirl to chop all fine. Beat in nutmeg and egg yolks. Beat egg whites with lemon juice until stiff. Fold beaten whites with spinach mixture. Spread 1 tablespoon tomato sauce in bottom of each of 3 soufflé dishes (1-pint size). Fill lightly with soufflé mixture. Level top with spatula, then run thumb around inside of each soufflé dish to form an indent in baking. Sprinkle tops with remaining 1 tablespoon Parmesan cheese. Bake at 450° F for 15 minutes. *Makes 3 servings, 130 calories per serving.*

Note: For varied soufflés, use broccoli or other vegetables in place of spinach.

16

Detailed Tips on Tasting Food Instead of Just _____Ingesting Food

You learned specifically in Chapter 5 *how to taste Deliciousness*—clearly and simply, with no complicated procedures—a great aid in slimming down and staying trim. We trust that you're using those recommendations and making them a foundation of your daily eating/living pattern. Basically you've acquired the essential knowledge of how to add and enjoy truly good taste in foods without consuming excess calories.

By following the D.D. ways of tasting and eating, you've lost your excess weight, according to your personal goal. Along similar relaxed and modified lines, you'll sustain your slim figure with Nutri-Maintenance Eating. The further Delicious stay-trim aids here and throughout this book will increase your enjoyment of living and eating—to help keep yourself in top physical condition.

You should be confident that you *can* change ingrown eating habits that lead to overweight; the success of millions of newly trim individuals with our methods proves it. Both D.D. techniques work in tandem: (1) with Delicious Dieting you take off excess weight; (2) Nutri-Maintenance Eating keeps you trim. Using both techniques alternately governs your choices daily and conditions you to good eating habits for life.

True gourmet food preparation today aims to *simplify* in order to bring out the pure flavors of fine foods that delight the taste and don't burden the digestion or encourage the storage of excess calories.

A scholar of gastronomy pointed out that the excesses of the past are out of tune with modern times. The drive now is to live *lean* to ensure a most attractive appearance, vigorous activity, and buoyant good health. He pointed out that in past centuries the so-called "aristocracy" demonstrated its superiority and wealth by overloading tables and bodies.

Chefs figured then that they manifested their ability not by cooking simply but by smothering foods with rich, heavy, complicated sauces that drowned out the good natural tastes. Many of royalty and power ate rich and fatty foods because they felt that being fat was a sign of being wealthy and powerful.

On the contrary, good eating today "purifies" food and delights the palate by eliminating what the famed three-star chef called "extraneous excretions." Nowadays overeating is a sign of *not* eating well; the true gourmet eats cleanly and selectively.

The focus of Delicious cooking, Delicious tasting, and Delicious eating is typified in statements by renowned French chefs Jean and Pierre Troisgros: "We respect the treasures of the earth. . . . Why damage or mask the flavor of fine meat, the verdant freshness of spring vegetables?" They favored "precise timing and delicate sauces divested of complication—to accompany, perhaps to exalt, but always to allow ingredients to be what they are."

The goal of Delicious Dieting and D.D. Nutri-Maintenance Eating, separately and combined, is to help you not only to eat most delectably but also most healthfully—to look and feel and *be* the best that you personally can be.

YOUR EVOLUTION TO BETTER TASTE

The D.D. dual system works logically, this way: If you've been conditioned from childhood to eat rich, greasy, high-calorie food, you've come to accept—without thinking about it—that a "rich" taste is good taste. Similarly, as you eat nongreasy food on Delicious Dieting and then on Nutri-Maintenance Eating, you've now become accustomed to enjoying purer, more naturally flavorful taste.

Like most people, after going through that unconscious transformation, you'll undoubtedly find that now you can't stand overly rich, high-calorie eating. Not only does such fatty food taste unpleasant, it tends to make you feel ill. But when you avoid them, you get the sustaining lift of increased vigor and well-being from eating more healthfully and certainly more deliciously.

Here are further Delicious stay-trim aids for better taste and better health.

1. *Live the difference between enjoying vs. engorging food.* When you devour greedily, you grow fat. When you choose carefully, eat slowly, and savor every mouthful, you *enjoy* every bit that you eat—and you stay lean and lovely. Tasting slowly is tasting fully—and that applies both to good food and good drink. To a hostess, it's a sign that guests *respect* what she is serving and what they are eating.

Many overweights who boast that they know and appreciate good food—which they cram down hastily, nevertheless—don't understand this scientific fact: *The stomach has no taste buds.* Your taste buds, "the end-organs of the sense of taste," are cells of the *tongue.* You taste and enjoy flavors in the mouth, not the stomach. If you gobble and gulp rapidly, you bypass the source of true flavor and taste. Certainly the stomach reacts, sometimes violently, to excesses of fat, sharp seasonings, and to other harmful elements in food—but the stomach cannot taste.

2. *Use "a touch of" instead of a lot.* To get the most from extra *flavor* without excess calories, use "a touch of" a high-calorie ingredient to improve taste discreetly. For example, "a touch of" milk, sweet butter, margarine, vegetable oil, sugar, and other ingredients can help keep you trim by enhancing your eating enjoyment without loading on unwanted pounds. An excess in *total* calories per day is the villain.

You'll note how this "touch of" taste bonus is provided in some of the Delicious Diet and Nutri-Maintenance recipes. But beware when servings are overloaded with these ingredients. A gentle touch in food preparation can enhance flavors and eliminate a ton of calories in the course of daily eating. Be cautious: if you think you may be adding too much of a high-calorie ingredient, then you are.

IMPROVE TASTE WITH
HERBS, SPICES, SEASONINGS

Take advantage too of "a touch of" additives that enhance flavor and texture with practically no calories. A little sometimes goes far. These include caraway seeds, poppy seeds, sesame seeds, a few flavorful capers (salty, but only about 6 calories per tablespoon), a sprinkle of grated Romano, Parmesan, or other hard, aged cheeses (to sparkle up vegetables, eggs, rice, pasta, and other foods).

Don't forget a squeeze of fresh lemon juice—either fresh or bottled. Lemon and lime add extra zing to many dishes and drinks.

Indeed, practically all herbs, spices, and seasonings can improve the taste of many servings and should become part of your daily food preparation with an eye on keeping calories low. But limit salt and sugar drastically for many health reasons as well as to keep weight from climbing.

Also add to your cooking and flavoring arsenal small amounts of zingy ingredients such as fresh ginger, onion flakes, minced onions, shallots, fresh chopped parsley. Check food store shelves for availability and ideas, and grow your favorites yourself on a windowsill or in a small garden space.

Refer to the following checklist for ideas when preparing and serving foods. None of these components add any significant calories to servings but can brighten up foods considerably.

CHECKLIST OF HERBS, SPICES, SEASONINGS

FOR POULTRY

Basil	Garlic	Oregano	Rosemary
Bay Leaves	Ginger	Paprika	Saffron
Cayenne	Marjoram	Parsley	Sage
Chervil	Mint	Pepper	Savory
Coriander	Mustard	Poultry Seasoning	Tarragon
Cumin	Onion		Thyme
Curry			

FOR FISH, SHELLFISH

Allspice	Curry	Marjoram	Rosemary
Bay Leaves	Dill	Mint	Sage
Cayenne	Fennel	Onion	Savory
Celery Seed	Garlic	Paprika	Thyme
Chervil	Ginger	Parsley	
	Mace		

FOR SALADS, VEGETABLES, EGGS

Cayenne	Dill	Paprika	Tarragon
Chervil	Garlic	Parsley	Thyme
Coriander	Ginger	Rosemary	
Cumin	Onion	Sage	
	Oregano		

CHECKLIST OF HERBS, SPICES, SEASONINGS

FOR MEAT

Allspice	Dill	Oregano	Rosemary
Basil	Garlic	Paprika	Sage
Bay Leaves	Ginger	Parsley	Savory
Chili	Marjoram	Pepper	Tarragon
Cloves	Mint	Red Pepper (Cay-	Thyme
Curry	Mustard	enne)	Tumeric
	Onion		

SAVING CALORIES AS YOU STEP UP TASTE

---

1. *When buying and preparing meat, keep in mind always that "lean" means comparatively clean of extra fat calories.* Insist that the butcher trim off sizable areas of visible fat—or do it yourself at home; you'll probably find more fat to remove even after the butcher has done his job.

Prepackaged meats are usually loaded with excess fat that you'll have to trim off. Be careful when shopping, for this may make a seemingly lower-priced package higher in the cost of the actual amount of meat you've bought.

Bypass stewing meats, which are generally higher in fat content. Veal and lamb usually contain less fat than beef, but check carefully, especially when buying lamb.

When buying chopped meat for hamburgers or meat loaf, beware of prepackaged "ground beef," which can contain up to 30 percent added fat, according to government regulations. Insist that lean chuck or top sirloin be ground to order for you (shop where this is done readily, or read the labels on prepackaged ground meats to find those labeled 80% lean, 20% fat).

Broil hamburgers rather than fry them. When you fry any kind of meat, not only are the fats usually added to the cooking surface beforehand (as in fast-food restaurants), but the *internal* fat is not removed; that's true even if you use a nonstick pan or vegetable cooking spray. Broiling removes a desirable amount of the internal fat, which drips off.

Another tip about hamburgers: Consider broiling lower-calorie chickenburgers, turkeyburgers, and vealburgers instead of beefburgers. Add flavor without calories to any hamburgers with herbs, spices, and other seasonings.

CAUTION: Speaking of hamburgers, and applying to any foods, we remind you again that "a touch of" adds flavor but "a ton of" the same ingredient can zoom the total calorie content. "A touch of" catsup, for example, smeared thinly on a lean, broiled hamburger or mixed in lean chopped meat doesn't add significant calories. But, if you eat even something like cottage cheese "drenched with catsup" (an astonishing favorite dish of an ex-President), you'd be adding up to 60 calories (3 tablespoons). Catsup contains plenty of sugar in the form of corn sweetener (check the label).

If a recipe calls for "larding" meat on the outside with fats or bacon, use plain cabbage leaves instead—you'll get the same cooking benefits without adding grease and calories.

Obviously, the more fat you cook out of meat, the more fat calories you eliminate. Therefore, well-done or medium-cooked meat has fewer calories than rare. On a 4-ounce piece of meat, "well done" is about 25 calories fewer than "rare." This is worth knowing, but as a matter of personal preference perhaps you'd settle for a smaller portion of rare steak or roast beef rather than a larger serving well done.

When cooking meats, chill the natural juices and then remove the fat (calories) after it rises and hardens. The natural fat-free meat juice, zipped up with a touch of lemon juice and even wine, makes a tasteful substitute instead of oil or mayonnaise in preparing meat salads and such.

You can save money and add delicious flavor by choosing cheaper cuts of lean meats and *marinating* them. The recipes for *D.D. French or Italian Salad Dressings or *D.D. No-Oil Dressing make excellent marinades. They'll become favorites of yours as you use them to tenderize meat and instill more delectable taste, but add practically no calories.

2. *A little wine, brandy, or even beer in small quantities adds subtle flavor and moistness to many recipes.* The alcohol is cooked away in the heating process and leaves better taste—with very few calories.

Use a dry (not sweet) wine, which contains less natural sugar and therefore fewer calories. A dry Chablis, domestic or imported, contains about 60 to 70 calories for a 3-ounce glass. But in cooking, after the alcohol evaporates, only 4 or 5 calories remain at most. For best taste results in cooking and basting, dry red wines are usually preferable for red meats—dry white wines are generally preferred in recipes for chicken, fish, shellfish, and veal.

205

Dry wine makes a desirable marinade since it adds a fine, subtle taste that enhances without intruding on good, natural flavor. Because of its high acid content, it helps to break down fibers and to tenderize cuts of less costly but tougher lean meats. Inexpensive wines are fine. "Cooking wines" may be used but often have high salt content—check the label.

3. *Use a little vinegar to pep up many dishes* such as stews, barbecued chicken and meats, fish, mixed vegetables, and salads. A tablespoon of cider or wine vinegar adds a lot of tangy flavor but only 2 or 3 calories.

4. *Remove fat from soups, gravies, meat and poultry juices*, and you remove greasy taste and fattening excess calories—while leaving clean, light flavor, better for your digestion and health. Here are some simple ways:

- With some recipes you can see the fat on top, so spoon it off while cooking and afterward.
- Refrigerate fat-containing food until fat rises to the top and hardens, then remove.
- For speedier fat removal, pour the liquid into a bowl. Add a few ice cubes, which will cause fat to rise to the top quickly—then just spoon off the fat and remove the ice cubes before they can dilute the flavor. Reheat the liquid, and serve.
- Here's a neat trick: Float a paper towel on top of the liquid for a few minutes. The towel will "attract" the fat so that when you lift off the piece, some of the fat comes with it, and you can now see and remove more fat with a spoon.

5. *Improve taste and avoid excess calories* by cutting out rich or greasy additives such as heavy gravies, sauces, and dressings that actually *deaden* delicious natural flavors. The different taste—and particularly the savings in calories—may be astonishing, as in these examples:

If you fry a fresh egg in a no-stick pan, or use a squirt of vegetable cooking spray—instead of adding a tablespoon of margarine, butter, oil, or other fat—*you'll save 100 calories*.

A substantial portion of broccoli, steamed to firm/tender perfection is only about 50 calories. But—if you add only 2 tablespoons of the usual Hollandaise sauce (very little to spoon on, isn't it?), you're loading on about *300 extra calories* to that serving of just one vegetable.

6. *Keep a D.D. high-flavor low-calorie dip in the refrigerator—* along with a variety of washed and cleaned celery stalks, carrot sticks, cauliflower buds, raw mushrooms, radishes, sweet pepper strips, arugula, and so on. Make sure the vegetables have their freshness and crispness preserved in a tightly covered container or damp towel. Enjoy the low-calorie treats as a snack or with a meal, enhanced by a quick stab into the tasty D.D. dip, if you like (see index for recipes).

7. *To enliven the salads you eat and serve,* select a variety of greens and lettuces, rather than just one. Fortunately supermarkets, farmers markets, and other stores are offering a greater selection now. In addition to the usual iceberg, Romaine, and Boston lettuces, look for arugula, Bibb, redleaf, and others.

Combine the lettuce with other greens and raw vegetables such as watercress, chicory, escarole, spinach, parsley, scallions, broccoli, cauliflower buds, green beans, snow peas, sugar snap peas, sweet red pepper, cherry tomatoes—the variety is almost endless. Add herbs and seasonings as you like. You'll find that the overall delicious taste is a combination of flavor, texture, and appealing shapes and colors, too.

8. *Note a few D.D. taste-improving tips to help you take off excess weight speedily and keep it off:*
- Be creative in preparing and serving vegetables. Often you can add appeal by combining vegetables—such as mushrooms and green beans, cooked tomatoes and pearl onions, spinach and okra. Let your imagination, and the availability of this produce, take it from there.
- It costs very little but can add a lot of flavor and sparkle when you have peppercorns in a grinder on the table, handy for cooking. Freshly ground pepper provides more zing than already ground pepper in a shaker. Such little touches can make a big difference in satisfying your taste without adding calories.
- Create your own personal herb/spice combinations. Don't overlook the fresh, added sparkle of dill when cooking many vegetables such as brussels sprouts, cabbage, spinach, and green beans. The natural flavor of fresh-picked tomatoes is brightened by a hint of basil in stewing. Try adding a little nutmeg when cooking green beans. Experiment with your own concoctions—it's fun and results in better taste.
- Be an artist in adding taste and eye appeal to servings with

colorful garnishes on the plate. Add the green leaves of watercress or airy, emerald sprays of parsley . . . carrots twisted into curls or cut in long thin sticks or chewy chunks . . . varicolored cucumber slices or spears . . . red and white radishes sculpted into rose petals with a paring knife. All that is Delicious creativity indeed.

- Chop, slice, shred, grate—with or without a food processor—to improve the taste of food through its *appearance*. You also change the actual taste of many foods this way. Consider how different it tastes when you nibble a long, very skinny julienned carrot strip—compared with chomping into an inch-thick carrot chunk. Many foods offer such opportunities. Add a few *chopped nuts* where fitting, for extra nutrition and flavor.

When eating out, as well as in preparing food at home, always be conscious of opportunities to cut calories and enjoy purer, natural taste at the same time. For instance, if you're tempted by Seafood à la Newburg on a menu or in a cookbook, realize that the thick, creamy, high-fat, high-calorie sauce loads your system with extra calories you don't want or need.

Consider a seafood and fish broil instead, flavored with a little wine, herbs, seasonings—then sparkled up with fresh lemon juice. You'll savor the delectable natural flavor of the fish itself— as you keep excess calories and fat from building bulges on your body.

You can elevate taste and lower calories throughout the meal. If you've decided on a bowl of soup for lunch, your taste buds will delight in a delicately seasoned, fat-free fresh vegetable soup rather than heavy beef-and-barley soup or frankfurter-and-lentil—as you eliminate *hundreds* of extra calories. For dessert, a fresh fruit cup enlivened with a little sparkling wine or a dash of liqueur is a gourmet treat—compared with a rich, creamy, sugary pastry totaling hundreds of calories. Stay aware of the many ways to preserve your newly slim, liberated (from overweight) body. Stop and think before reverting to the outmoded habits of food preparation and selection that overwhelmed you with excess pounds and inches in the past. Be observant and creative.

- To provide delicious variety in salads, use clear gelatin molds at times, made more delectable by substituting vegetable juice, tomato juice, fruit juice, broth—instead of water. As the filling in the gelatin mold, cubed leftover cooked vegetables, raw vegetables, cut-up fruits, chicken, turkey, shellfish, fresh or canned fish, and lean meats are a few of the possibilities.

- When serving relatively low-calorie hot soups for lunch, especially during cold weather, enhance the flavor to make each spoonful taste "special." Possibilities are endless with a little creative thinking. Here are a few ideas that please the palate and are nutritious and satisfying:

  . . . Start with clear chicken consommé, or fat-free chicken broth with rice or noodles. Add cubes of leftover chicken if available, or pieces of vegetables such as green beans and carrots. When the soup has just started to simmer, gently stir in a well-beaten egg. Top the steaming soup in the bowl with a few sprinkles of grated Parmesan cheese and chopped parsley or chives.

  . . . Heat fat-free Manhattan clam chowder (no milk or cream), add a few teaspoons of chopped chives and several tablespoons of chopped clams or whole baby clams. Sprinkle in one or two of your favorite herbs. At the point of simmering, add a tablespoon of white wine or light sherry, let simmer but not boil for a few minutes. It's delicious, and the few wine calories will have simmered away.

  . . . In a pan of fat-free onion or tomato soup, sprinkle some chopped watercress, chopped parsley, or chives. Stir in a tablespoon of grated sharp cheddar or Romano cheese. Simmer for a few minutes. Serve with a couple of sesame breadsticks or your favorite low-calorie crispbread or crackers—there are many on the market.

- Don't overlook pineapple to pep up many salads and other foods, thus adding much flavor but surprisingly few calories. Because pineapple is naturally so sweet, many people jump to the conclusion that it's high in calories. When it's fresh or packed in its own juice—*no sugar added*—pineapple has about 70 calories per ½ cup, but if you add sugar or it's packed in heavy syrup, the calorie count zooms. Because of the full flavor, only a few chunks of pineapple provide luscious extra flavor in salads, fruit cups, varied vegetable combinations, and other mixes.

- Instead of reaching from habit for sour cream and heavy cream to add to your shopping basket, consider all the delicious ways you can substitute low-fat yogurt and low fat cottage cheese. Combine the cottage cheese in a blender with a little skim milk, perhaps a touch of lemon juice, a few herbs—for a "sour cream" alternate that saves hundreds of calories while providing light, fresh taste.

- Extend the use of foods such as canned salmon by combining them in a blender with herbs and low-fat cottage cheese. You'll find this mixture delicious and money-saving for salads or open sandwiches served on Melba toast or other low-calorie breads and crackers. Don't be tempted to add mayonnaise!

- As a midmorning, midafternoon, or evening snack, consider a mug of hot broth transformed into a zesty, attractive, and satisfying concoction. As one example, combine in a pan some plain tomato juice, fat-free chicken or beef broth, lemon juice, and a dash of curry powder, ground nutmeg, or cinnamon. Heat to a simmer, pour into a mug, and top with a sprinkle of chopped parsley or chives. Add a thin slice of lemon into which you've inserted several cloves. Hearty, attractive, sustaining.

Summing up: Be alert to the many ways of creativity in cooking, plus calorie- and taste- consciousness, and you'll achieve your goal—*never heavy again*—by maintaining D.D. simple, practicable basics.

17

Activity Plan to Aid Speediest Reducing and Lifelong Top Vigor—Fitting Your Personal Lifestyle

There's no question that keeping your body active and moving can be a definite help in slimming down and staying trim. We strongly recommend *activity* as a vital health and fitness aid. That means moving your body meaningfully according to your personal desires and abilities. It does not mean trying to become a muscle-bound athlete. It encompasses anything that fits you, from walking briskly to more demanding programs.

Just don't expect activity or sports alone to take off any sizable amount of excess weight. It won't work.

Movement specialist Jane Boutelle in her book *Lifetime Fitness for Women* (which I co-authored) stresses that basic point, emanating from her lifelong experience in successfully conditioning women and men of all ages. She states that activity and exercise are excellent and essential to "trim off inches by tightening and firming loose, sagging muscles that support the bones—*but to reduce overweight, you must diet.*"

Recent scientific findings indicate that there may be impressive dual benefits from a sustained activity session that stimulates the individual's metabolism. First, it is universally agreed that exercising the body burns up many more calories than being sedentary and still. Secondly, and less well known, the prolonged-activity period results in burning more calories for as much as *hours* after the extended movement session.

Some people still think that activity and action tend to increase the appetite and thus interfere with weight loss. There is growing scientific opinion to the contrary—that activity and exercise help diminish rather than boost the appetite. We're not aware of incontrovertible evidence on either side. In any case, when you eat the D.D. way, controlling your appetite becomes relatively pleasant, and the pounds vanish speedily.

Since sustained movement brings considerable benefits, we urge you to be *active*. So . . . what activity is best for you, to go along with your Delicious Dieting, in trimming inches and pounds away?

Becoming physically fit should and can be enjoyable, not a grind or a chore. Your rule: Do, but don't overdo. There's danger in plunging into overly exhausting activity. Don't be like the extremist who overexercises desperately and winds up gasping, "I'm going to make myself fit even if it kills me!"

Sensible, moderate activity such as brisk walking, swimming, bicycling—in that order—are the most recommended pursuits for the average person, according to medical consensus. Amateur and professional athletes are in a separate category that doesn't concern us here; they are usually guided by knowledgeable trainers and coaches.

Your fundamental purpose is to attain maximum fitness within your personal desires, capacities, and limitations. "Fitness implies the ability to withstand the emergency demands of everyday living," according to Dr. Warren R. Guild, former associate in medicine at Harvard Medical School and member of the President's Council on Physical Fitness. He noted, "People sleep better, think better, digest better, enjoy more, and feel better when they are in shape."

Your body was built for *movement*, to keep going at top individual effectiveness. The right conditioning provides a wonderful bonus: Your joy in living increases emphatically when you look and feel in shape and take pride in your newly acquired appearance. That springs from a combination of slimming down to your desired weight and steady use of your body for at least 15 to 20 minutes of prolonged movement daily.

Caution again: Do, but don't overdo. Please keep in mind Jane Boutelle's advice that you undertake "smooth-running, rhythmic natural actions contrasting with overstraining manipulations" in whatever you do. She warns, "I have always been opposed to the dangerous but still prevalent concept that 'It's not doing you any good unless it hurts.' Realize that it's *how* you move that counts, not how fast or how hard you move. My firm rule is that

212

if you ever feel the slightest pain or strain, tell yourself instantly, 'Whoa, stop, that's enough'—and rest before you go on, or try again tomorrow.'' We endorse that caution for you totally.

WHAT ACTIVITY IS BEST FOR YOU?

This is not an "exercise book"—there are plenty of excellent volumes around for you to consult. What we offer here is a consensus of current medical opinion about generally effective and safe activity for the average person. Make your choices according to your personal likes—and get approval from your physician before undertaking any strenuous program.

BREATHING MOST PRODUCTIVELY

Breathing correctly and effectively should be part of any activity program, and can boost your energy and fitness with every breath. Yet it's estimated that as many as 90 percent of us don't know how to breathe properly.

Briefly: With correct, full deep breathing, you inhale and breathe in oxygen through your nose . . . you exhale and breathe out carbon dioxide. Breathing properly for maximum health rewards can as much as double *vital lung capacity* for many. Boosting your supply of oxygen helps your system burn up food and calories most effectively, aids in promoting desirable weight loss—along with improving your health as a whole.

Correct breathing is simple, pleasant, energizing. It becomes natural with practice. We recommend this slow in-out breathing session first thing in the morning, and repeatedly during the day and evening when convenient. It's this easy:

One: Standing or sitting, breathe in slowly and deeply through your nose . . . as you raise your stiffened arms directly forward from your sides to straight up overhead—and hold in the air as long as comfortable.

Two: Purse your lips and breathe out through your mouth very s-l-o-w-l-y, as though you're blowing a long note through a bugle—while lowering your stiffened arms slowly in the same forward parallel movement to your sides where you started.

Repeat this one-two action up to 15 times, being careful not to become breathless. If you feel any strain, *stop*. With this slow, measured breathing, you'll get an energizing boost. It will become part of your improved physical conditioning and functioning. You can be pleased that you'll be helping your calories-IN calories-OUT stay-trim equation every day.

BRISK WALKING

The emphasis here is decidedly *not* on sauntering or strolling, but on *brisk* walking. Certainly dawdling can be pleasant and rewarding as you admire the passing scene and the beauties of nature, out in the open air. However, don't expect to get much benefit physically that way. You must use your muscles meaningfully for at least twenty minutes.

That energetic (not rushing or straining) sustained movement of your legs, arms, and body improves circulation and helps to build new "roadways" for smoother blood flow to and from your heart muscle. Your lungs take in more oxygen to feed your moving muscles. The prolonged action helps to firm muscles and work your feet and the entire length of your legs—beneficially affecting your ankles, calves, knees, thighs, hips, buttocks, abdomen, and diaphragm.

No, you shouldn't race along or strain with exaggerated emphasis. Wear comfortable shoes and clothing, of course. Move smoothly, conscious of your legs, arms, and other parts of your body in invigorating action. Walk "tall," not slouched or stooped, and without stress.

Be aware of pulling in your stomach muscles comfortably, chest up, back straight but not as stiff as a board, shoulders up but relaxed, head and neck erect but not strained. Move your legs primarily from the hips, not the knees. Inhale and exhale deeply and smoothly, not jerkily. *It's important—walking, standing, sitting—to be posture conscious this way; it helps you appear slimmer, by flattening your abdomen (abdomIN) and thus flattering your figure; you feel better about yourself emotionally as well as physically.*

Of course, as you walk along in sustained fashion, you pause for traffic and other necessities. Then you move ahead again smoothly, keeping the rhythm going for about twenty minutes or half an hour or more, as time and your sense of enjoyment allow. If you care to dig deeper into the subject, read a book on walking.

Grasp opportunities for walking as they occur, being aware of the possibilities. Instead of hopping into your car or a taxi for a short ride, perhaps you can walk. Consider using stairs to go up a floor or two, rather than automatically stepping into an elevator.

PROLONGED-ACTION SWIMMING

Swimming is excellent health-building, health-sustaining body conditioning as well as enjoyable recreation. But dunking in the water, wading about with a brief spurt here and a backfloat there, won't do you much physical good. That should be called "bathing" rather than "swimming."

Get your pleasure from being in and near the water, of course, but realize that stop-and-go (mostly stop) "swimming" isn't real body-toning exercise. Smooth-flowing prolonged-action rhythm does the most for you; avoid pushing, pulling, puffing, gasping, and general overexertion.

To gain the greatest benefit for your heart, lungs, and total muscular structure, get into the habit of prolonged-action swimming on a regular basis—daily if you can, but at least three times a week for half an hour or more. You may wish to team up with others who have learned the benefits of swimming laps.

Don't race or push yourself beyond comfortable endurance. If you need to pause for a few minutes, keep moving—*bob up and down* slowly and rhythmically for a few minutes as you hold onto a ladder, grip the side of the pool, or stand in shallow water. Flex your knees slightly with the movement, breathing deeply but effortlessly.

Lap swimming is part of an effective fitness program for increasing numbers of people of all ages. Within weeks you'll find yourself enjoying and reaping all sorts of physical and emotional benefits. We've seen it work wonders for posture and general vigor. Coupled with your Delicious Diet and D.D. Nutri-Maintenance Eating, you'll find that you're trimming inches off thighs and hips, flattening your abdomen, and slimming off excess pounds beautifully.

PROLONGED-ACTION BICYCLING

Bicycling is another potentially effective conditioning exercise when done with prolonged-action movement. If you just dawdle along on your bike, letting the wheels do most of the work—with your legs and joints limply following along automatically—you'll get recreational and social pleasure but very little physical benefit.

If you move with conscious effort, without straining or jerking, pumping your legs vigorously and smoothly, and you *keep going* that way for twenty minutes or more (pausing for traffic and such, if necessary), you'll be improving your physique, increasing your bloodflow desirably, and using up calories. Just be aware that if you meander down the road on your bike, drifting, stopping to chat with friends, you'll be kidding yourself if you say, "I've had my exercise for today, been for a nice spin on my bike."

A special advantage of bicycling for body conditioning is that you can do it indoors as well—with a stationary bicycle, motorized or not. As a lifelong participant in all-over body movement for physical conditioning, I strongly recommend my proven method of "TV watcher's exercising." As a professional writer, working at my typewriter much of the day, I maintain top muscle tone and physical conditioning this way:

I have a motorized exercise-bicycle against a wall in my study (previously in the bedroom), from which I have a direct view of the TV screen on a portable set. I find that riding my stationary bike, or jogging in place, doing calisthenics, or using a rowing machine for twenty minutes is boring unless my attention is fixed on the screen. You may prefer to exercise while listening to the radio, records, or cassettes.

I turn on whatever I find acceptable on one of the stations, and watch as I move my body vigorously on the exercise bike. My leg muscles benefit exceptionally as they work *against* the motorized circling pedals, resisting their forward action. I bend, stretch, and breathe deeply. By raising and lowering the handlebars every other minute, I can shift the position of my body—sitting erect, then bending from the hips.

I enjoy three twenty-minute prolonged-action sessions per day—about two hours after early breakfast (following an hour or more at the typewriter), then just before lunch, and the third session in early evening after a long day of sedentary deskwork. In addition, I exercise my body first thing in the morning for a ten-minute period of natural actions, mostly on my back on the bathroom floor; same in a hotel room if traveling. I add a similar workout in the evening before bedtime.

I've pursued this schedule for the past twenty years (wearing out two exercise bicycles), and when I have my annual checkup by our longtime physician, the doctor invariably commends my good muscle tone, slimness, limberness, continuing strong heart action. . . . "Great, keep doing what you're doing, stay slim and keep your body moving."

You can do the same indoors if you wish, selecting whatever kind of program pleases you most. Choose from walking or jogging in place, using a stationary bike, rowing machine, other exercise apparatus, or a calisthenics method—whatever suits you personally.

A recent Cornell University study suggests that the body burns off more calories when you exercise *within two to three hours after a meal* (but not immediately after eating). These researchers stress further that *regularity* in exercising is more important than *intensity* of activity. The key to maximum benefit is prolonged action for twenty minutes or more daily (as little as a brisk, continuous twenty-minute walk), or for as many days a week as fits your lifestyle.

Try "TV watcher's exercising" yourself as a regular movement program. Even if you dislike most TV programming, you'll always find something on the screen you can enjoy or tolerate or despise (see how the other half lives). Don't say, "I haven't time for exercising," since you can be conditioning your body and working off calories instead of sitting in front of the TV or listening to radio, records, or cassettes.

We guarantee that keeping your body in motion is a lot healthier, and definitely more slimming, than sitting passively and exercising your hand by digging into a bowl of potato chips.

JOGGING . . . RUNNING . . . SPORTS

Jogging and running can be effective body conditioning in many ways—*if done with forethought and understanding.* Foot and leg injuries are likely to occur when an individual overdoes, or plunges haphazardly into these demanding activities without needed preparation and equipment, such as proper supportive shoes. We urge that you first get approval from your doctor, then read a sound book on jogging and running, and seek advice from experts and experienced joggers.

The same caution is true for strenuous sports such as tennis, in which intelligent preparation and warmup procedures provide some protection against too-common injuries. Similarly, if you wish to undertake weightlifting, judo, and yoga, get qualified information and advice beforehand—and be sure the methods don't exceed your personal capacities and goals.

Use your good sense to realize that some sports do supply desirable body conditioning with reasonable vigor and prolonged action, but others are more for recreational pleasure and don't activate the body sufficiently for sustained physical benefits.

Examples of prolonged-action sports include sustained walking/hiking, bicycling, tennis, table tennis, squash, rowing, canoeing, and cross-country skiing. Sports that are fine hobbies, providing recreation and mental relaxation but not much sustained action, include golf (not so relaxing if you have a short fuse), sailing, motorboating, hunting, and fishing. Enjoy them, of course, but understand the need for prolonged-action endeavors as well.

EXERCISE CLASSES

Millions get body-conditioning benefits from properly planned exercise classes. A poorly run physical conditioning method, whether amateur or professional, can involve injurious movements that may seriously damage the back and other parts of the body.

Ask everyone you know for recommendations. Then it's best to watch and try a sample class before joining an extended course. A couple of hour-long classes a week in an effective program can be a great boon for correct body alignment and posture, neuromuscular (nerve and muscular systems) toning and coordination, and neuromuscular stamina and endurance.

Machines and weights may or may not be used; basically your body alone is the best "machine" for improving your health and physical well-being. It is also beneficial to combine classes with supplementary periods of body movement at home; the course instructor may have the needed information in a book or pamphlet for expanding the same actions at home.

CALORIES-OUT CHART

There's no point in you personally trying to figure out how many calories you expend every time you take a brisk walk or indulge in a sport or simply chew your food, sit, or sleep. It's certainly not necessary, since you lose weight swiftly on your Delicious Diet without counting calories.

Nevertheless, as a matter of interest, if your mind runs along mathematical or investigative lines (are you a crossword puzzle addict?), you might be curious to note how many calories are generally used up in various activities, as shown on the following chart.

Experts agree that the average person should expend a minimum of 300 to 500 calories daily in activity. We must emphasize again that you can't count on exercise alone as a significant weight-loss method. Citing weight training as an example, a health researcher stated that "caloric expenditure in a twenty-minute weight workout is the equivalent of about eight potato chips."

In another instance, when questioned on a TV talk show about the physical demands and weight-reduction possibilities of sexual intercourse, a doctor we know explained, "Well . . . performing the sex act does get rid of some calories, but if you eat a small apple afterwards, that will replace all the calories you've expended." Hmmmm.

In checking the figures here, bear in mind that these are general and approximate assessments and can't possibly be applied accurately to every individual. Your weight, age, and how much you personally tend to exert in each action—such as how vigorously you move—all influence your caloric output. All considered, here's a broad-range checklist:

APPROXIMATE CALORIC EXPENDITURES FOR A HALF-HOUR PERIOD
Activity/Exercise/Common Procedures

APPROXIMATE CALORIC EXPENDITURE	120-LB. WOMAN	160- LB. MAN
Badminton	180–220	220–260
Baseball	160–200	200–240
Basketball	300–400	400–600
Bicycling (energetic)	200–230	280–320
Bicycling (moderate)	100–120	120–140
Bowling	80–120	100–140

APPROXIMATE CALORIC EXPENDITURES FOR A HALF-HOUR PERIOD
Activity/Exercise/Common Procedures

APPROXIMATE CALORIC EXPENDITURE	120-LB. WOMAN	160- LB. MAN
Canoeing	100–150	130–180
Carpentry (workbench)	120–140	140–180
Climbing stairs	130–160	160–190
Cooking (active)	60–90	80–110
Dancing (energetic)	200–400	250–500
Dancing (moderate)	100–130	130–170
Dishwashing (by hand)	60–90	80–110
Dressing, undressing	30–50	35–60
Driving auto	50–60	60–75
Dusting (energetic)	80–100	80–110
Eating slowly, chewing	40–50	50–80
Exercising (energetic)	200–250	250–350
Exercising (moderate)	140–170	180–220
Fencing	110–130	130–160
Football	250–300	300–400
Gardening (active)	120–140	140–180
Golf (no cart)	100–140	130–170
Golf (with cart)	70–90	80–110
Handball	200–350	300–400
Hockey (field, ice)	250–300	300–400
Horseback riding	140–160	160–200
Housework (active)	80–130	110–160
Ironing	60–80	70–90
Jogging (light)	200–250	250–300
Karate	320–350	360–400
Lacrosse	250–300	350–400
Laundering (moderate)	50–70	70–90
Lawn mowing (hand mower)	100–130	130–150
Lawn mowing (power mower)	90–110	110–140
Lying, sitting, at rest	15–20	20–25
Office work (active)	70–130	90–150
Painting walls, furniture	130–150	150–180
Piano playing	80–130	100–150
Polishing furniture, auto	80–120	90–150
Reading	15–20	20–25
Rowing (vigorous)	300–400	400–500
Running	300–400	400–500
Sawing wood	250–300	300–400
Sewing, knitting, crocheting	30–40	40–60
Singing	35–40	40–60
Skating (energetic)	200–300	250–350
Skiing (energetic)	200–300	250–350
Sleeping	25–30	30–40
Square dancing	140–160	160–180

APPROXIMATE CALORIC EXPENDITURES FOR A HALF-HOUR PERIOD
Activity/Exercise/Common Procedures

APPROXIMATE CALORIC EXPENDITURE	120-LB. WOMAN	160-LB. MAN
Soccer	250–300	350–400
Squash	180–240	250–400
Standing (relaxed)	20–25	25–30
Sweeping floor	80–100	90–110
Swimming (sustained)	200–300	300–400
Table tennis	150–180	200–250
Tennis (amateur)	180–220	250–280
TV viewing	25–30	30–40
Typing	80–100	90–110
Vacuuming	120–140	140–160
Violin playing	70–100	90–130
Volleyball	180–220	220–280
Walking (energetic)	140–160	160–180
Walking (moderate)	80–100	90–120
Water skiing	210–230	230–250
Writing	25–80	30–100

ABOVE ALL . . . ENJOY!

Please don't let yourself get fanatical about your body conditioning. As with dieting, if you miss a day or two or more, don't worry about it. Start over again and take pleasure in your activity, along with getting the benefits you want and need.

You'll profit lifelong from the great partnership of weight control through D.D. stay-trim eating and prolonged-action body conditioning. This union works: Managing calories-IN healthfully through Delicious Dieting and Nutri-Maintenance Eating . . . plus boosting calories-OUT with effective physical movement on a day-in, day-out basis.

The union provides stronger, more enduring health and all-over fitness than dieting or exercising alone. The result is akin to entwining two strands of thin rope into a cable—that multiplies the strength of the cable far beyond the capacity of each strand individually.

Your uplifting, enduring reward as you become slimmer and trimmer is that you not only look and feel better, but also you *move* better—more gracefully, more beautifully. That's a most worthy and fulfilling goal!

18

Valuable Added Data to Slim Down and Stay Trim

Food Contents Checklist:
Calories, Protein,
Fat, Carbohydrates

The information in this chapter is for your convenient reference, as a helpful but not essential aid in taking off pounds and inches—and keeping them off. That's the specific purpose of this book, not just to help you reduce swiftly, healthfully, and beautifully, but to provide the clear, simple means for staying trim lifelong.

Skim through the listings for the large variety of foods now, if you like—to get an overall idea of the facts and how they may be helpful to your personal needs. Then you'll probably find yourself returning repeatedly to the detailed data for checking purposes. The material here is by no means a complete compendium of nutritional information. Also, the figures listed are subject to some variations. Obviously, each cut of chicken, meat, or fish, every piece of fruit or vegetable, and other types of foods—differ to some extent in composition, texture, and other common variables. For your purposes, the general calorie and other counts are sufficiently dependable to use as a basic measure.

It's nonproductive to become obsessed about counting calories—like Snoopy, the dog in the "Peanuts" comic strip, trying to find out for his bird friends the number of calories in a single bread crumb. If you find yourself comparing different calorie and contents tables, don't be concerned if the counts fluctuate a few calories more or less per item.

It's the total calories per day over a succession of days that matter in maintaining desired weight. A small number of calories alone isn't significant. As stressed earlier, your true guide is your morning weigh-in on the scale. That number tells you specifically whether you are losing, maintaining, or gaining weight.

As you are now thoroughly aware, you don't count calories on the Delicious Quick-Trim Diets. At times, you may find it helpful and enlightening to refer to the numbers of calories, protein, fat, and carbohydrates (C-P-F-C). Thus you can readily check items as an aid in making personal choices, especially in maintenance eating.

This can guide your decisions in selecting what to buy or prepare in your home or to choose from a menu in a restaurant. You discover in seconds, for example, that a 3½-ounce serving of lean steak provides about 200 calories, a little more than 30 grams of protein, 7 grams of fat, and no carbohydrates. Comparably, a 3½-ounce portion of broiled halibut amounts to about 170 calories, 25 grams of protein, 7 grams of fat, and no carbohydrates.

If you're choosing fruit for breakfast or any meal, it's instructive to read that half a cantaloupe, 5 inches in diameter, contains 40 calories, 1 gram of protein, only a trace of fat, and 9 grams of carbohydrates. For purposes of comparison again, a cup of blueberries supplies about 90 calories, 1 gram of protein, 1 gram of fat, and 19 grams of carbohydrates. Thus, you know instantly that half a cup of blueberries has about the same C-P-F-C as half a cantaloupe. You can make a reasoned selection accordingly.

Much of the data on these pages is based on the excellent handbook *Composition of Foods*, produced by the Agricultural Research Service of the United States Department of Agriculture. Cross-checks have been made with other sources. Copies of the sizable USDA handbook, totaling close to 200 pages, are obtainable at very reasonable cost from the Superintendent of Documents, U.S. Government Printing Office, Washington, DC 20402.

MEASUREMENTS GUIDE

BY WEIGHT:
1 ounce equals 28.35 grams
100 grams equal 3.57 ounces
16 ounces equal 1 pound

BY VOLUME CAPACITY:
1 cup equals 8 fluid ounces or ½ pint or 16 tablespoons
1 tablespoon equals 3 teaspoons
2 tablespoons equal 1 fluid ounce
1 pint equals 2 cups
1 quart equals 4 cups

FOOD CONTENTS CHECKLIST
Calories . . Protein . . Fat . . Carbohydrates

Appearing here in the following sequence:
- Poultry and Meats
- Fish and Shellfish
- Vegetables
- Fruits and Fruit Products
- Milk, Cheese, Eggs, Related Foods
- Fats, Oils, Shortenings
- Grain Products: Breads, Cereals, Cakes, Grains
- Sweets, Sugar, Nuts
- Beverages
- Soups, Jams, Miscellaneous

FOODS: PORTION	CALORIES	PROTEIN *(grams)*	FAT *(grams)*	CARBO-HYDRATES *(grams)*
POULTRY AND MEATS				
Bacon, crisp, drained, thin-sliced: 2 slices	95	5	8	1
Bacon, Canadian, crisp, drained, trimmed: 1 oz.	79	8	5	trace
Beef, trimmed, cooked:				
Braised, simmered, pot-roasted:				
lean and fat: 3½ oz.	286	27	19	0
lean only: 3½ oz.	196	31	7	0
Hamburger, broiled:				
regular market ground:				
3½ oz.	286	24.5	20	0
ground lean: 3½ oz.	216	27	11.5	0
Rib, or other relatively fat roast, oven-cooked without liquid:				
lean and fat: 3½ oz.	455	19	42	0
lean only: 3½ oz.	233	27	14	0
Round, or other relatively lean cut:				
lean and fat: 3½ oz.	256	27	16	0
lean only: 3½ oz.	182	29	5.5	0
Steak, broiled: relatively fat, such as sirloin				
lean and fat: 3½ oz.	385	23	31.5	0
lean only: 3½ oz.	201	31.5	7	0

FOODS: PORTION	CALORIES	PROTEIN (grams)	FAT (grams)	CARBO- HYDRATES (grams)
Porterhouse:				
57% lean, 43% fat: 3½ oz.	465	19.5	42	0
separable lean: 3½ oz.	224	30	10.5	0
T-Bone:				
56% lean, 44% fat: 3½ oz	473	19.5	43	0
separable lean: 3½ oz.	223	30	10	0
Club steak:				
58% lean, 42% fat: 3½ oz.	454	20.5	40.5	0
separable lean: 3½ oz.	244	29.5	13	0
Beef, corned beef:				
cooked, medium fat: 3½ oz.	372	23	30	0
canned lean: 3½ oz.	185	26	8	0
Beef, dried or chipped: 2 oz.	372	23	30	0
Beef liver, fried: 3½ oz.	229	26	10.5	5.5
cooked without fat (or raw):				
3½ oz.	140	20	4	5.5
Beef Tongue:				
cooked, braised: 3½ oz.	244	21.5	17	0
canned or pickled: 3½ oz.	267	19	20	trace
Chicken; cooked:				
Broilers:				
flesh and skin, broiled,				
without bone: 3½ oz.	216	28	11	0
light meat, without skin:				
3½ oz.	166	31.5	3.5	0
dark meat, without skin:				
3½ oz.	176	28	6	0
Roasters:				
flesh and skin, roasted:				
3½ oz.	248	27	14.5	0
flesh only, roasted: 3½ oz.	183	29.5	6	0
canned, boneless: 3½ oz.	170	25	7	0
Livers, simmered: 3½ oz.	165	26.5	4.5	3
Duck; domestic, roasted:				
4 oz.	370	18	32	0
Goose, domestic, roasted:				
4 oz.	480	27	42	0
Lamb:				
Leg (choice grade): total edible, cooked, roasted (83% lean, 17% fat):				
3½ oz.	279	25	19	0
separable lean, roasted:				
3½ oz.	186	28.5	7	0

FOODS: PORTION	CALORIES	PROTEIN (grams)	FAT (grams)	CARBO- HYDRATES (grams)
Loin (choice grade): total edible, broiled chops (72% lean, 25% fat): 3½ oz.	293	16.5	25	0
separable lean, broiled chops: 3½ oz.	188	28	7.5	0
Shoulder (choice grade): cooked, roasted (74% lean, 26% fat): 3½ oz.	338	21.5	27	0
separable lean: 3½ oz.	205	27	10	0
Pork, fresh: Composite of trimmed, lean cuts: ham, loin, shoulder, and spareribs:				
medium fat class, cooked, roasted (77% lean, 23% fat): 3½ oz.	373	22.5	30.5	0
separable lean: 3½ oz.	236	28	13	0
Chop, thick, with bone: 3½ oz.	260	16	21	0
Chop, lean only: 1.7 oz.	130	15	7	0
Roast, oven-cooked, no liquid added:				
lean and fat: 3 oz.	310	21	24	0
lean only: 2.4 oz.	175	20	10	0
Pork, cured:				
Ham, medium-fat:				
cooked, roasted, (84% lean, 16% fat): 3½ oz.	289	21	22	0
separable lean: 3½ oz.	187	25	9	0
canned: 3½ oz.	287	18	12	1
Picnic:				
cooked, roasted (82% lean, 18% fat): 3½ oz.	323	22.5	25	0
separable lean: 3½ oz.	211	28.5	10	0
Rabbit, cooked, stewed: 3½ oz.	216	29	10	0
Sausage, cold cuts, and luncheon meats:				
Bologna (average): 3½ oz.	277	13.5	23	3.5
Braunschweiger: 3½ oz.	319	15	27.5	2.5
Cervelat (soft): 3½ oz.	307	18.5	24.5	1.5
Country-style sausage: 3½ oz.	345	15	31	0
Deviled ham, canned: 3½ oz.	351	14	32.5	0
Frankfurters, cooked: 3½ oz.	304	12.5	27	1.5
Liverwurst, smoked: 3½ oz.	319	15	27.5	2.5

FOODS: PORTION	CALORIES	PROTEIN (grams)	FAT (grams)	CARBO-HYDRATES (grams)
Luncheon meat:				
Boiled ham: 3½ oz.	234	19	17	0
Pork Sausage, links or bulk,				
cooked: 3½ oz.	476	18	44	trace
Salami, dry: 3½ oz.	450	24	38	1
Sweetbreads:				
Beef, cooked: 3½ oz.	320	26	23	0
Calf, cooked: 3½ oz.	168	32.5	3	0
Lamb, cooked: 3½ oz.	175	28	6	0
Turkey:				
total edible, cooked, roasted:				
3½ oz.	263	27	16.5	0
flesh and skin, roasted: 3½ oz.	223	32	9.5	0
flesh only, cooked, roasted:				
3½ oz.	190	31.5	6	0
light meat, cooked, roasted:				
3½ oz.	176	33	4	0
dark meat, cooked, roasted:				
3½ oz.	203	30	8.5	0
Veal:				
average cut, medium fat,				
trimmed, roasted (86%				
lean, 14% fat): 3½ oz.	216	28.5	10.5	0
cutlet, broiled without bone:				
3 oz.	185	23	9	4
FISH AND SHELLFISH				
Anchovy, canned: 3 fillets	21	2.5	1	trace
Bass, black sea:				
poached, broiled, or baked				
without fat: 3½ oz.	93	19	1	0
Bass, striped raw: 3½ oz.	105	19	2.5	0
Bluefish, raw: 3½ oz.	117	20.5	3.5	0
Clams, raw, meat only: 3½ oz.	76	12.5	1.5	2
canned, drained: 3½ oz.	98	16	2.5	2
juice: 3½ oz.	19	2.5	trace	2
Cod, cooked or broiled: 3½ oz.	170	28.5	5.5	0
dried, salted: 3½ oz.	130	29	1	0
Crab, Dungeness, rock, and				
King, cooked, steamed:				
3½ oz.	93	17.5	2	.5
Fish sticks, frozen, cooked:				
3½ oz.	176	16.5	9	6.5

FOODS: PORTION	CALORIES	PROTEIN *(grams)*	FAT *(grams)*	CARBO-HYDRATES *(grams)*
Flounder, raw: 3½ oz.	79	16.5	1	0
Haddock, raw: 3½ oz.	79	18.5	trace	0
Halibut, Atlantic & Pacific, cooked, broiled: 3½ oz.	171	25	7	0
Herring, raw:				
Atlantic: 3½ oz.	176	17.5	11.5	0
Pacific: 3½ oz.	98	17.5	2.5	0
canned, tomato sauce: 3½ oz.	176	16	10.5	3.5
pickled: 3½ oz.	223	20.5	15	0
salted or brined: 3½ oz.	218	19	15	0
kippered: 3½ oz.	211	22	13	0
Lobster, northern, canned or cooked: 3½ oz.	95	19	1.5	.5
Mackerel, canned: 3½ oz.	183	19.5	11	0
salted: 3½ oz.	305	18.5	25	0
smoked: 3½ oz.	219	24	13	0
Mussels, meat only: 3½ oz.	95	14.5	2	3.5
Ocean perch (redfish): 3½ oz.	88	18	1	0
Octopus, raw: 3½ oz.	73	15.5	1	0
Oysters, raw:				
Eastern: 3½ oz.	66	8.5	2	3.5
Western: 3½ oz.	91	10.5	2	6.5
Oysters, fried: 3½ oz.	239	8.5	14	18.5
Pike, broiled: 3½ oz.	90	19	1	0
Pompano, raw: 3½ oz.	166	19	9.5	0
Red Snapper (and gray) raw: 3½ oz.	93	20	1	0
Salmon, Atlantic, raw: 3½ oz.	217	22.5	13.5	0
canned, solids and liquids: 3½ oz.	203	21.5	12	0
Chinook (King), raw: 3½ oz.	222	19	15.5	0
canned, solids and liquids: 3½ oz.	210	19.5	14	0
Coho, canned, solids and liquids: 3½ oz.	153	21	7	0
cooked, broiled, or baked: 3½ oz.	182	27	7.5	0
smoked: 3½ oz.	176	21.5	9.5	0
Sardines, drained solids: 3¾ oz.	190	18	12.5	1.5
Scallops, bay and sea:				
cooked, steamed: 3½ oz.	112	23	1.5	—
frozen, breaded, fried, reheated: 3½ oz.	194	18	8.5	10.5
Seabass, white, raw: 3½ oz.	96	21.5	.5	0

FOODS: PORTION	CALORIES	PROTEIN (grams)	FAT (grams)	CARBO-HYDRATES (grams)
Shad, raw: 3½ oz.	170	18.5	10	0
Shrimp, canned, meat only:				
3½ oz.	116	24	1	1
French fried: 3½ oz.	225	20.5	11	10
Smelts, 4–5, raw:	100	19	2	0
Sole, raw (also flounder,				
sandcrabs): 3½ oz.	79	16.5	1	0
Swordfish, raw: 3½ oz.	118	19	4	0
Trout, brook, raw:				
3½ oz.	101	19	2	0
rainbow or steelhead, raw				
3½ oz.	195	21.5	11.5	0
Tuna, canned in oil:				
solids and liquid: 3½ oz.	288	24	20.5	0
drained solids: 3½ oz.	197	29	8	0
canned in water: 3½ oz.	127	28	1	0
Weakfish, raw: 3½ oz.	121	16.5	5.5	0
Whitefish, lake, raw: 3½ oz.	155	19	8	0
smoked: 3½ oz.	155	20	7.5	0
VEGETABLES				
Artichoke, cooked: 3½ oz.	44	3	trace	10
Artichoke hearts, frozen: 3 oz.	22	1	trace	4
Asparagus, med. spear, canned:	3	trace	trace	.5
6 spears	20	2	trace	3
Avocado, large: ½	180	2	16.5	6
Bamboo shoots, raw: 3½ oz.	27	2.5	trace	5
Bean sprouts:				
cooked (mung beans): 1 cup	28	3	trace	5
raw: 1 cup	26	3	trace	4
Bean sprouts (soy bean): 1 cup	50	7	1	5
Beans, green, cooked: 1 cup	25	2	trace	6
wax, cooked: 1 cup	22	1.5	trace	4.5
lima (green), cooked: 1 cup	197	13	1	35
dry lima, cooked: 1 cup	265	15.5	1	49
red kidney, cooked: 1 cup	234	15	1	42.5
Beets, diced: 1 cup	70	2	trace	16
Broccoli: 1 cup	50	5	trace	8
Brussels sprouts,				
cooked: 1 cup	50	5.5	.5	8.5
Cabbage, raw, shredded: 1 cup	25	1	trace	5
cooked: 1 cup	40	2	trace	9
Cabbage (Chinese cabbage):				
raw 1" pieces: 1 cup	15	1	trace	2
cooked: 1 cup	25	2	1	4

FOODS: PORTION	CALORIES	PROTEIN (grams)	FAT (grams)	CARBO-HYDRATES (grams)
Carrots, 5½", raw: 1 cup	20	1	trace	5
diced: 1 cup	45	1	1	9
Cauliflower, cooked, flowerbuds: 1 cup	30	3	trace	6
Celery, 8" stalk, raw:	5	1	trace	1
diced, cooked: 1 cup	20	1	trace	4
Chard, Swiss, cooked: 1 cup	30	2.7	.3	5
Chick-peas, dry, raw: ½ cup	360	20	4.5	60
Chives, chopped, fresh: 1 tbs.	3	.2	0	.5
Collards, leaves, cooked: 1 cup	65	7	1.3	10
Corn, cooked, 5" ear	65	2	1	16
canned, with liquid: 1 cup	170	5	1	41
Cucumber, 1 med. raw:	16	1	trace	3
6⅛" center slices	5	trace	trace	1
pickle, sweet, 1 med.	146	.5	trace	36.5
pickle, sour or dill: 1 large	11	.5	trace	22
Eggplant, cooked: 1 cup	34	2	trace	7
Endive, fresh: 1 cup	10	1	trace	2
(escarole, chicory) Belgian Endive, 4": 1	5	trace	trace	1
Kale, cooked: 1 cup	45	4	1	8
Kohlrabi, cooked: 1 cup	36	2.5	trace	8
Leeks, raw: 1 cup	104	4	.5	22
Lentils, cooked: 1 cup	212	15.5	trace	39.5
Lettuce, headed, fresh:				
loose leaf, 4" diam.: 1 head	30	3	trace	6
compact, 4¾" diam.: 1 head	70	4	.5	12.5
2 large or 4 small leaves	5	1	trace	trace
Mushrooms, cooked or canned: 1 cup	41	4.5	trace	5.5
Okra, cooked: 8 pods	30	2	trace	6
Olives,				
green: 1 large	9	trace	1	trace
ripe: 1 large	13	trace	1.5	trace
Onions, mature:				
raw, 2½" diam.: 1 onion	50	2	trace	11
cooked: 1 cup	80	2	trace	18
Onions, young green, small, no tops: 6 onions	25	trace	trace	5
Parsley, fresh, chopped: 1 tbs.	1	trace	trace	trace
Parsnips, cooked: 1 cup	95	2	1	22
Peas, green:				
cooked: 1 cup	110	8	1	19
canned, with liquid: 1 cup	170	8	1	32

FOODS: PORTION	CALORIES	PROTEIN (grams)	FAT (grams)	CARBO-HYDRATES (grams)
Peppers,				
sweet, green: 1 medium	15	1	trace	3
red: 1 pod	20	1	trace	3
Potatoes, med. (about 3 lbs.):				
baked, after peeling: 1 potato	90	3	trace	21
boiled, peeled after boiling: 1				
potato	105	3	trace	23
boiled, peeled before boiling: 1				
potato	90	3	trace	21
French fried, 1 piece 2″ × ½″				
× ½″: 10 pieces	155	2	7	20
chips, medium, 2″ diam.: 10				
chips	110	1	7	10
mashed (with milk added): 1				
cup	145	4	1	30
Pumpkin, canned: 1 cup	83	2	1	18
Radishes, small: 4	10	trace	trace	2
Rutabagas, cooked,				
diced: 1 cup	70	1.8	.2	16
Sauerkraut, canned, drained: 1				
cup	30	2	trace	6
Soybeans, mature, cooked: 1 cup	277	22	11.5	21.5
immature, raw	284	22	10	26
Spinach, cooked: 1 cup	45	6	1	6
Squash, cooked:				
summer, diced: 1 cup	35	1	trace	8
winter, baked, mashed: 1 cup	126	3	.5	30
summer, raw: 1 cup	38	2	trace	8
Sweet Potatoes:				
baked (1 sweet potato 5″ × 2″)	155	2	1	36
boiled (1 sweet potato 5″ × 2″)	170	2	1	39
candied (1 sweet potato 3½″ ×				
2¼″)	295	2	6	60
Tomatoes:				
fresh, 1 medium 2″ × 2½″	30	2	trace	6
canned, or cooked: 1 cup	45	2	trace	9
Tomato juice, canned: 1 cup	50	2	trace	9
Tomato catsup: 1 tbs.	15	trace	trace	4
Turnips, cooked, diced: 1 cup	40	1	trace	9
Vegetable juice, cocktail, canned				
or bottled: 6 oz.	31	1.5	trace	6.5
Water chestnuts, Chinese, fresh: 4				
average	20	trace	trace	4.5
Watercress: 1 cup	10	1	trace	1.5

FOODS: PORTION	CALORIES	PROTEIN (grams)	FAT (grams)	CARBO-HYDRATES (grams)
FRUITS AND FRUIT PRODUCTS				
Apples, fresh: 1 medium (2½" diam.)	70	trace	trace	18
Applesauce, fresh: 1 cup	125	trace	0	32
Applesauce, canned:				
sweetened: 1 cup	185	trace	trace	47
unsweetened: 1 cup	100	trace	trace	25
Apple juice, cider: 4 oz.	52	trace	0	12.5
Apricots, fresh, 12 per lb.: 3	60	1	trace	14
canned in heavy syrup: 1 cup	218	1.5	trace	53
dried, uncooked, 40 halves, small: 1 cup	390	7.5	1	89
cooked, unsweetened, fruit and liquid: 1 cup	260	5	1	62
nectar: 1 cup	143	1	trace	34
Banana, fresh, about 3 per lb.: 1	130	2	trace	30.5
Blackberries, fresh: 1 cup	85	2	1	17
Blueberries, fresh: 1 cup	89	1	1	19
Cantaloupe, fresh: ½ melon, 5" diam.	40	1	trace	9
Cherries:				
fresh, sour: 1 cup	116	2	0.5	25
fresh, sweet: 1 cup	140	2.5	.5	32
Cranberries:				
canned sauce, sweetened, strained: 1 cup	400	trace	.5	99
Juice, cocktail, canned: 1 cup	130	trace	trace	32
Cranberry-Orange relish, fresh: 3½ oz.	178	trace	trace	45
Dates, dried, pitted: 1 medium	27	trace	trace	6.5
1 cup	525	4	1	120
Elderberries, fresh: ½ cup	70	2.5	trace	16
Figs, dried, 2" × 1": 1 fig	60	1	trace	15
Fruit cocktail, canned, in heavy syrup (with liquid): 1 cup	195	1	trace	47
Gooseberries, fresh: ½ cup	88	1.8	.5	20
Grapefruit, fresh, med., 4½" diam.:				
½ fruit	50	1	trace	12
fresh sections: 1 cup	75	1	trace	18
canned, water pack: 1 cup	70	1	trace	17
juice, fresh: 1 cup	95	1	trace	23
canned:				
unsweetened: 1 cup	100	1	trace	24
sweetened: 1 cup	130	1	trace	32

FOODS: PORTION	CALORIES	PROTEIN (grams)	FAT (grams)	CARBO-HYDRATES (grams)
frozen concentrate, water				
added: 1 cup	115	1	trace	28
Grapes, fresh, green:				
seedless, 1 cup	102	1	trace	27
other (approx.): 1 cup	100	1	trace	26
Grape juice, bottled: 1 cup	165	1	trace	42
Lemons, fresh, 2⅓" diam.:				
1 lemon	20	1	trace	6
juice: 1 tbs.	5	trace	trace	1
Lemonade concentrate, water				
added: 1 cup	110	trace	trace	28
Lime juice, fresh: 1 tbs.	4	trace	trace	1
Limeade concentrate, water				
added: 1 cup	103	trace	trace	26
Mandarin oranges, canned wtih				
syrup: 1 cup	125	1	.5	30
Mango, fresh, edible parts: ½ lb.	155	1.5	1	35
dried or sliced: ½ cup: 2½ oz.	53	.5	.3	12
Nectarine, fresh: 1 med.	50	.5	trace	12
Orange, fresh:				
navel, California, 2⅘" diam:				
1 orange	60	2	trace	13
others, 3" diam.: 1 orange	70	1	trace	17
Orange juice, fresh:				
California: 1 cup	120	2	1	26
Florida: 1 cup	100	1	trace	23
canned, unsweetened: 1 cup	120	2	trace	28
frozen concentrate, water				
added: 1 cup	110	2	trace	26
Papaya, fresh, ½" cubes: 1 cup	71	1	trace	17
1 large	156	2	trace	38
Peaches, fresh, medium:				
2" diam. (4 per lb): 1 peach	33	.5	trace	8
sliced: 1 cup	65	1	trace	16
canned, heavy syrup: 2				
halves, 2 tbs. syrup	96	trace	trace	24
water pack: 1 cup	75	1	trace	19
Peach nectar, canned: 1 cup	124	trace	trace	31
Pears, fresh (3" × 2½" diam.):				
1 pear	100	1	1	24
canned in heavy syrup, halves				
or slices: 1 cup	200	1	trace	50
canned, water packed: 1 cup	80	trace	trace	20

233

FOODS: PORTION	CALORIES	PROTEIN *(grams)*	FAT *(grams)*	CARBO-HYDRATES *(grams)*
Pear Nectar, canned: 1 cup	130	1	trace	33
Persimmons, Japanese or Kaki,				
fresh, 2½" diam.: 1	80	1	trace	20
Pineapple				
fresh, diced: 1 cup	75	1	trace	19
canned in syrup, crushed:				
1 cup	205	1	trace	50
sliced (slices and juice): 2 sm.	95	trace	trace	25
canned, packed in own syrup:				
3½ oz.	58	trace	trace	15
Pineapple juice, canned: 1 cup	120	1	trace	31
Plums (not prunes):				
fresh, 2" diam., about 2 oz.:				
1 plum	30	trace	trace	7
canned in syrup: 3 plums,				
2 tbs. juice	90	trace	trace	23
Prunes, dried:				
medium, 50 or 60 per lb: 4	80	1	trace	19
cooked, unsweetened, 17–18				
prunes and ⅓ cup liquid:				
1 cup	330	3	1	80
Prune juice, canned: 1 cup	185	1	trace	42
Raisins, dried: 1 cup	462	4	trace	111
Raspberries, red, fresh: 1 cup	70	1	.5	16
frozen, sweetened: 1 cup	196	1.5	trace	47
Rhubarb, cooked, sugar added:				
1 cup	385	1	trace	98
Strawberries, fresh: 1 cup	55	1	1	11
frozen, sliced, sweetened: 1				
cup	247	1	trace	60
Tangerines, fresh 2½" diam.,				
about 4 per lb.: 1	40	1	trace	10
Tangerine juice, canned:				
unsweetened: 1 cup	105	1	trace	25
frozen, water added: 1 cup	115	1	trace	27
Watermelon, fresh: 4" × 8"				
wedge	240	4.5	2	52
balls or cubes: 1 cup	56	1	trace	12

MILK, CHEESE, EGGS, RELATED FOODS
Cheese (1 ounce except where
  otherwise noted)

American	106	6	9	.5

FOODS: PORTION	CALORIES	PROTEIN (grams)	FAT (grams)	CARBO-HYDRATES (grams)
American Pimiento	106	6	9	.5
Blue	100	6	8	.5
Brie	95	6	8	trace
Camembert	85	6	7	trace
Cheddar	114	7	9.5	.5
Cottage, creamed: ½ cup	117	14	5	3.5
uncreamed: ½ cup	96	19.5	.5	2
pot cheese, low-fat 2% fat:				
½ cup	101	15.5	2	4
pot cheese, low-fat, 1% fat:				
½ cup	82	14	1	3
Cream	99	2	10	1
Edam	101	7	8	.5
Feta	75	4	6	1
Fontina	110	7	9	.5
Gouda	101	7	8	.5
Limburger	93	6	8	trace
Monterey	106	7.0	8.5	trace
Mozzarella	80	5.5	6	.5
Mozzarella, part skim	72	7	4.5	1
Muenster	104	6.5	8.5	.5
Neufchâtel	74	3	6.5	1
Parmesan, grated:	111	10	7.5	1
1 tbs.	23	2	1.5	trace
Port du Salut	100	6.5	8	trace
Ricotta: ½ cup	216	14	16	4
Ricotta, part skim: ½ cup	171	14	10	6.5
Romano	110	9	7.5	1.0
Roquefort	105	6	8.5	.5
Swiss:				
natural, domestic	107	8	7.5	4.0
processed	95	7	7	.5
Cheese food, American	94	5.5	7	2.5
Cheese spread, American	82	4.5	6.0	2.5
Cream: 1 tbs.				
half and half	20	.5	1.5	.5
light, table, or coffee	29	.5	3	.5
medium (25% fat)	37	.5	4	.5
sour	26	.5	2.5	.5
sour, imitation, cultured	20	.5	2	.5
whipping cream topping	8	trace	1	.5
whipping, heavy, whipped	26	trace	3	trace
whipping, heavy, unwhipped	52	.5	5.5	.5

FOODS: PORTION	CALORIES	PROTEIN (grams)	FAT (grams)	CARBO-HYDRATES (grams)
whipping, light, whipped	22	trace	2.5	trace
whipping, light, unwhipped	44	.5	4.5	.5
Creamer:				
liquid, frozen: ½ oz.	20	trace	2.0	1.5
nondairy, powder: 1 tsp.	11	trace	1	1
Milk, canned, undiluted: 1 fl. oz.				
condensed, sweetened	123	3.0	3.5	21
evaporated, whole,				
unsweetened: 1 fl. oz.	42	2	2.5	3
evaporated, skim, canned:				
1 fl. oz.	25	2.5	trace	3.5
milk, dry, skim:				
nonfat solids: ¼ cup	109	11	trace	15.5
whole	159	8.5	8.5	12.5
fresh (1 cup): 8 fl oz:				
buttermilk, cultured, skim	99	8	2	12
skim	86	8.5	.5	12
skimmed partially, 1% fat	102	8.0	2.5	11.5
skimmed partially, 2% fat	125	8.5	4.5	12
whole, 3.7% fat	157	8.0	.9	11.5
Yogurt, plain, low-fat: 1 cup	120	8.0	4.0	13
whole milk: 1 cup	139	8	7.5	10.5
Eggs, chicken, raw or cooked				
without fat				
white only from 1 large egg	16	3.5	trace	.5
whole, 1 large	79	6	5.5	.5
yolk only from 1 large egg	63	3	5.5	trace
Eggs, dried, whole: 2 tbs.	60	4.5	4	.5
FATS, OILS, SHORTENINGS				
Butter, 4 sticks per lb.				
2 sticks = 1 cup	1,626	2	184	trace
⅛ stick = 1 tbs.	100	trace	11	trace
1 pat (90 per lb.)	36	trace	4	trace
Fats, cooking:				
bacon fat, chicken fat: 1 tbs.	126	0	14	0
lard: 1 cup	1,985	1	220	0
1 tbs.	124	0	14	0
margarine, 4 sticks per lb.				
2 sticks = 1 cup	1,633	1.5	183	1
⅛ stick = 1 tbs.	102	trace	11	trace
1 pat (80 per lb.)	36	trace	4	trace

FOODS: PORTION	CALORIES	PROTEIN (grams)	FAT (grams)	CARBO-HYDRATES (grams)
Oils, salad or cooking:				
corn, cottonseed, olive,				
soybean, peanut,				
safflower oils: 1 tbs.	125	0	14	0
Salad dressings:				
blue cheese: 1 tbs.	90	1	10	.5
imitation mayonnaise type: 1				
tbs.	60	trace	6	2
French: 1 tbs.	60	trace	6	2
mayonnaise: 1 tbs.	110	trace	12	trace
Thousand island: 1 tbs.	75	trace	8	1

GRAIN PRODUCTS: BREADS, CEREALS, CAKES, GRAINS

FOODS: PORTION	CALORIES	PROTEIN (grams)	FAT (grams)	CARBO-HYDRATES (grams)
Barley, pearled, uncooked: 1 cup	782	18	2	173
Biscuits, baking powder				
2½" diam.: 1 biscuit	138	3	6.5	17
Bran flakes (40% bran): 1 oz.	87	3	.5	18
Breads:				
cracked wheat (20 slices per				
lb.): 1 slice	60	2	1	12
French, enriched: 1 slice	58	2	1	11
Italian, enriched: 1 slice	55	2	.5	11
protein: 1 slice	45	2.5	0	8.5
pumpernickel, dark: 1 slice	56	2	trace	12
raisin (20 per loaf): 1 slice	60	2	1	12
rye, light: 1 slice	55	2	trace	12
white, enriched (20 per lb.): 1				
slice	60	2	1	12
(26 per lb.): 1 slice	45	1	1	9
whole wheat, graham all-				
wheat bread (20 per lb.):				
1 slice	55	2	1	11
Breadcrumbs, dry, grated: 1 cup	345	11	4	65
Cakes:				
angel food cake: 2" sector of 8"				
cake	110	3	trace	23
chocolate, fudge: 2" section of				
10" cake	420	5	14	70
fruitcake, dark 2" × 2" × ½":				
1 piece	105	2	4	17
gingerbread, 2" × 2" × 2":				
1 piece	180	2	7	28

FOODS: PORTION	CALORIES	PROTEIN (grams)	FAT (grams)	CARBO-HYDRATES (grams)
cupcake, plain, 2³/₄" diam.: 1 cake	160	3	3	31
pound cake, 2¾" × 3" × ⅝": slice	130	2	7	16
sponge, 2" sector, 8" diam. cake: 1 sector	115	3	2	22
Cookies:				
plain and assorted 3" diam.: 1 cookie	110	2	3	19
fig bars, small: 1	55	1	1	12
Corn flakes, enriched: 1 cup	93	2	trace	21
plain: 1 oz.	110	2	trace	24
presweetened: 1 oz.	115	1	trace	26
Cornmeal, white or yellow, dry: 1 cup	420	11	5	87
Corn muffins, 2¾" diameter: 1	155	4	5	22
Corn, puffed, presweetened, enriched: 1 oz.	100	1	trace	26
Crackers:				
graham: 4 small or 2 medium	55	1	1	10
saltines, 2" square: 2 crackers	35	1	1	6
soda, plain, 2½" square: 2 crackers	45	1	1	8
Crackermeal: 1 tbs.	45	1	1	7
Doughnuts, cake type: 1	135	2	7	17
Farina, enriched, cooked: 1 cup	105	3	trace	22
Macaroni, cooked until tender: 1 cup	155	5	1	32
Melba toast: 1 slice	15	.5	trace	2.5
Muffin, with enriched white flour: 2¾" diam.	135	4	5	19
Noodles (egg) cooked, enriched: 1 cup	200	7	2	37
Oatmeal or rolled oats, cooked: 1 cup	150	5	3	26
Pancakes, 4" diam.: 1 cake	60	2	2	8
buckwheat: 1 cake	45	2	2	6
Piecrust, enriched, 9" crust: 1 crust	655	10	36	72
Pie, 4" sector of 9" diam.:				
apple; cherry: 1 sector	330	3	13	53
custard: 1 sector	265	7	11	34
lemon meringue: 1 sector	300	4	12	45
mince: 1 sector	340	3	9	62

FOODS: PORTION	CALORIES	PROTEIN (grams)	FAT (grams)	CARBO-HYDRATES (grams)
pumpkin: 1 sector	265	5	12	34
Pizza (cheese), 5½" sector, ⅛ of 14" pie: 1 sector	180	8	6	23
Popcorn, popped: 1 cup	55	2	1	11
Rice, cooked:				
parboiled: 1 cup	205	4	trace	45
white: 1 cup	200	4	trace	44
Rice, puffed, enriched: 1 cup	55	1	trace	12
Rice flakes, enriched: 1 cup	115	2	trace	26
Rolls, 12 per pound: 1 roll	115	3	2	20
hard, round, 2 oz. ea.: 1 roll	160	5	2	31
Rye wafers, 1⅞" × 3½": 2 wafers	45	2	trace	10
Spaghetti, cooked until tender:				
1 cup	155	5	1	32
Wheat, puffed, enriched: 1 oz.	100	4	trace	22
presweetened: 1 oz.	105	1	trace	26
Wheat, shredded, plain: 1 oz.	100	4	.5	21
Wheat flakes: 1 oz.	100	3	trace	23
Wheat flours:				
whole wheat: 1 cup	420	16	2	85
all-purpose sifted: 1 cup	400	12	1	84
self-rising: 1 cup	385	10	1	81
Wheat germ: 1 tbs.	24	12	.5	2.5
SWEETS, SUGAR, NUTS				
Almonds, shelled: 1 cup	900	26	77	28
Brazil nuts, broken pieces: 1 cup	970	20	92	15
Candy:				
caramels: 1 oz.	120	1	3	22
chocolate, sweetened, milk:				
1 oz.	151	2	9	16
fudge, plain: 1 oz.	115	trace	3	23
hard candy: 1 oz.	110	0	0	28
marshmallow: 1 oz.	95	1	0	23
Cashew nuts, roasted: 1 cup	570	15	45	26
Coconut, dried, shredded,				
sweetened: 1 oz.	156	1	11	15
Gelatin, dry, plain: 1 tbs.	35	9	trace	0
Gelatin dessert, prepared:				
plain: 1 cup	155	4	trace	36
with fruit: 1 cup	180	3	trace	42
Peanuts, roasted, shelled:				
halves: 1 cup	885	37	69	29

FOODS: PORTION	CALORIES	PROTEIN (grams)	FAT (grams)	CARBO-HYDRATES (grams)
chopped: 1 tbs.	52	2	4	2
Peanut butter: 1 tbs.	93	4	8	3
Pecans:				
halves: 1 cup	760	10	74	15
chopped: 1 tbs.	50	1	5	1
Sherbet: 1 cup	235	3	trace	58
Sugar: 1 oz.	110	0	0	28
Walnuts, chopped: 1 cup	790	17	73	18
1 tbs.	50	1	4.5	1

BEVERAGES
Alcoholic:

FOODS: PORTION	CALORIES	PROTEIN (grams)	FAT (grams)	CARBO-HYDRATES (grams)
Beer, canned or bottled:				
regular: 12 fl oz.	150	1	0	12.5
low calorie: 12 fl oz.	under 100	1	0	3
*Distilled liquor: unflavored bourbon, brandy, Canadian whiskey, gin, Irish whiskey, Scotch whiskey, rum, rye whiskey, tequila, vodka:				
1 fl oz.	65–82*	0	0	trace
Wines:				
dessert (18.8% alcohol):				
3 oz.	117	trace	0	6.5
dry (12.2% alcohol): 3 oz.	75	trace	0	3.5
Carbonated (nonalcoholic):				
sweetened (quinine sodas):				
8 oz.	71	0	0	18
unsweetened (club soda)	0	0	0	0
cola type: 8 oz.	89	0	0	23
flavored sodas:				
sweetened: 8 oz.	105	0	0	27
unsweetened (diet soda):				
8 oz.	—	—	—	—
ginger ale, pale dry and				
golden: 8 oz.	71	—	—	18
root beer: 8 oz.	94	—	—	24
Coffee: 1 cup	2	trace	trace	.5
Tea: 1 cup	2	trace	trace	.5

*Calories average 70 for 86 proof; may vary up or down as indicated if higher or lower proof.

FOODS: PORTION	CALORIES	PROTEIN (grams)	FAT (grams)	CARBO-HYDRATES (grams)
SOUPS, JAMS, MISCELLANEOUS				
Bouillon cube, ⅝": 1	5	2	trace	trace
Bouillon mix, for 1 cup	10	2	trace	trace
Catsup, tomato: 1 tbs.	19	trace	trace	4.5
Chili sauce (mostly tomatoes):				
1 tbs.	15	trace	trace	4
Chocolate:				
bitter or unsweetened: 1 oz.	144	3	17.5	8
sweetened: 1 oz.	151	1	10	16.5
Chocolate syrup: 1 tbs.	40	trace	trace	11
Hollandaise sauce: 1 tbs.	48	1	4	2
Honey, strained or extracted:				
1 tbs.	64	trace	0	17
Jams, marmalades, preserves:				
1 tbs.	55	trace	trace	14
Jellies: 1 tbs.	50	0	0	13
Soups, canned, ready to serve:				
bean: 1 cup	190	8	5	30
beef: 1 cup	100	6	4	11
bouillon, broth, consommé:				
1 cup	10	2	—	0
clam chowder: 1 cup	85	5	2	12
cream soup (asparagus, celery,				
mushroom): 1 cup	200	7	12	18
noodle, rice, barley: 1 cup	115	6	4	13
pea: 1 cup	140	6	2	25
tomato (with water): 1 cup	86	2	2	15
vegetable: 1 cup	80	5	2	10
Syrup, table blends: 1 tbs.	55	0	0	15
Sugar, granulated, cane, or beet:				
1 cup	770	0	0	199
1 tbs.	48	0	0	12
lump, 1⅛" × ⅝" × ⅛": 1 lump	25	0	0	7
powdered (stirred up): 1 cup	495	0	0	127
brown, firm-packed: 1 cup	820	0	0	210
1 tbs.	51	0	0	13
Vinegar: 1 tbs.	2	0	0	1
White Sauce, medium: 1 cup	430	10	33	23

NOTE: If you wish to check any foods and beverages that don't appear in the listing here, you may find the data in the USDA *Compositions of Foods* handbook mentioned earlier, or elsewhere in your library.

19

Clear Answers to Dieters' Most-Asked Questions

Here are some straightforward answers to the questions most often asked of us by overweights during our combined fifty-plus years in the fields of health, diet, nutrition, and food preparation. We've been particularly gratified to be able to help overweight women and men to reduce most effectively and pleasantly, and to stay trim ever after. The direct, explicit answers—in no special order of importance—should aid you too.

Some of the questions have been answered previously in this book. Since repetition strengthens remembrance, these reminders, translated necessarily into action by *you*, can be most valuable in your program to reduce quickly and to stay trim lifelong. These composites of information have definitely helped other dieters—and now they're yours for the using.

"Is the Delicious Quick-Trim Diet guaranteed to reduce me?"

Yes, if you are in normal health, go on the Delicious Diet of your choice, and follow instructions precisely. No, if you don't go on the diet and stick with it, or if you deviate from directions considerably. Just owning the book and not using it according to D.D. Guidelines won't reduce you—sorry. But having read the book, obviously eager and willing to give Delicious Dieting a try, you can't miss. Eventual congratulations on your newly slim figure!

"Is the FAT in foods I eat the villain in making and keeping me overweight? . . . Don't the calories in the protein and carbohydrate contents contribute too?"

It's easy to figure that out for yourself according to comparative calorie contents: A gram of protein contains 4.4 calories . . . a gram of fat carries 9 calories . . . a gram of carbohydrate contributes 4 calories. Clearly, every ounce of fat in the food adds more than *twice the calories* of an ounce of protein or carbohydrate. That's a prime indicator of why Delicious Diets are very low in fat, helping to keep your total day's calorie intake down, taking off pounds and inches rapidly.

Sure, practically everything you eat adds calories, and it's the total excess calories per day that make one heavy. It's significant, however, that fatty foods are right at the top of the list of offenders—along with overconsumption of sweets. The moral: Eat according to D.D. guidelines and you'll be following the healthful, low-calorie, Quick-Trim way that means you'll reduce in a hurry and soon achieve and maintain the slim, trim body you desire.

> *"I'm determined to reduce from my ungainly 175 pounds to 120 pounds, to be slim and more attractive and active. I've been warned that my husband and friends may be jealous and upset about the change. What should I do?"*

Your good health and favorable self-image are far more important than any concern about possible upset or jealousy on the part of others—which probably won't happen. Those who really care about you will be delighted by your improvement and triumph. Your husband—if he is like most—will find you more attractive and exciting. Any others who might be envious or negative about the benefits you've achieved are hardly worth worrying about, right?

> *"How can I refuse gracefully when a hostess piles too much food on my plate or presses second helpings on me—and I don't want to insult her by refusing?"*

You should never be ungracious, offend your hostess, or make her uncomfortable by demanding special foods. Here are some alternatives to consider that make good sense and are in good taste:

"I've become a small eater—I'll enjoy every bit of this delicious food, but a little instead of a lot."

"Just a little, please—doctor's orders. Nothing serious, but I must lose weight."

"This is so delicious. I'll enjoy every bite. I don't need big portions to appreciate what you serve."

If a hostess pouts, "It's no fun feeding you," you might respond, "Sorry, everything looks great, but it's no fun being overweight—I'll look forward to eating more when I'm down to what I should weigh for my health and well-being."

"The food looks wonderful, but I'd rather come back for seconds than leave good food on my plate and waste it."

No hostess would try to force forbidden servings on a diabetic or others with health disabilities such as intense allergies. Nor would she insist that guests consume certain foods or excessive amounts that might make them ill. Similarly, intelligent hostesses and hosts don't press food or drinks on reluctant guests who are reducing or determined to stay trim. If they do bear down on you regardless, are you sure they are friends?

> *"Ever since I can remember, my mother kept stuffing food into me, insisting that being fat is being healthy. I'm afraid that I'm conditioned to being overweight, against my wishes. How can I overcome that conditioning?"*

Here are just three approaches you can consider and try:

1. You can decide that you're not a child anymore, but an adult responsible for your personal well-being and actions. Go on the Delicious Diet, stay with it, and you'll prove to yourself in a few days that you can lose weight—regardless of any inbred overeating habits.
2. If you haven't the gumption to diet, see a qualified psychologist or other therapist who may be able to help you to overcome this hangup.
3. If you still feel you can't diet, and won't consider therapy, decide to live with being overweight and continue to respect yourself.

> *"How many dress sizes can I drop on D.D.?"*

That depends on how overweight you are at the start, also your height and general figure conformation. Many women lose up to four dress sizes and even more. It's not uncommon to go from size 18 to 12 or even to 10. Delicious size-trimming indeed!

> *"I've never had any desire to eat at breakfast, just a cup of coffee—then I enjoy an early lunch and dinner. Will that pattern interfere with quick reducing on my Delicious Diet?"*

Keep to that eating pattern if you like, and ignore hidebound "experts" who insist on everyone having a "hearty breakfast" even if it loads on excess pounds. We're interested in helping you to slim down beautifully, not in sustaining rigid rules and regulations. Space out the foods on D.D. menus as you like. Just don't exceed the total specified intake for the day.

In fact, you'll lose weight even more swiftly if you divide the day's food into six feedings instead of three. Enjoy what you eat on D.D. when you feel like eating it.

"I plan to serve a Delicious Diet menu at a dinner party next week—shall I tell the guests that it's a low-calorie D.D. meal?"

We suggest that you not say anything about it until after dinner—after you've heard the compliments about how wonderful the food is. Then inform them or not, as you please. Unfortunately, many people have a closed mind about diets and think "low-calorie" or "diet" food can't possibly taste good. Your D.D. servings will prove otherwise, but let them learn for themselves. Thus you'll prevent them from letting their prejudices get in the way of their eating judgment and enjoyment.

"A very heavy friend said that when she tried a diet a few years ago, and had to give up rich food and sweets, she developed daily headaches. I'm afraid that will happen to me— what can I do about it?"

The first thing to do is to stop worrying and start Delicious Dieting. Your friend's headaches were probably psychologically induced. Feeling that she was depriving herself, and that her body needed the rich foods, the headaches occurred due to an imbalance in her system—in her view. One dieter said that she feared she'd get headaches because her body needed a lot of sugar; when it was pointed out that she'd get lots of sugar in the form of fructose from all the fruit on D.D., the headaches never occurred.

Most such "deprivation headaches" or "hunger headaches" stem from imagination and concern arising from resentment over the self-denial. It usually helps to realize that when you're overweight and cut rich foods, empty sweets, and empty calories, your body feeds on its own fat healthfully, thus trimming off pounds and inches. Many newly slim individuals have told us that their headaches vanished when they realized this.

Concentrate on how much lovelier and healthier you'll be rather than on any problems you fear might arise. If you should feel ill in any way, headaches or anything else, stop dieting until you check with a doctor and get the okay to proceed again. If you ever suffer repeatedly from headaches, see your doctor immediately, since this may be a symptom of serious illness.

"I heard a nutritionist say on the radio that if you have a great craving for a certain food, it means that your body needs it. Is that true?"

We too heard a "nutritionist" with doubtful credentials tell a caller on a radio advice program that if she had a craving for oranges it meant that her body needed vitamin C. When the listener said that her craving was for candy bars, she was told, "No, that's making an emotional demand, not a food or vitamin demand."

We recommend that you stick to your healthful, varied Delicious Diet until you're down to your desired weight. Then, when you're slim, you can satisfy a craving for a candy bar—which is not sinful. Please reread Nutri-Maintenance instructions.

"I fell off my diet, had a slice of chocolate layer cake, and feel terrible about it. What shall I do?"

Get right up and climb back on your diet again. Like everyone else, you're human and fallible, so don't waste time feeling guilty. Make up for it by following D.D. directions precisely from now on. As pounds fall off swiftly, you'll feel so good about it that you'll be less likely to slip off your diet again.

"Should I take vitamins on the Delicious Diet?"

As noted in D.D. instructions, the menus and variety of Delicious foods supply sufficient vitamins and minerals for adults in normal health. If you wish to take a multiple vitamin-mineral addition, that's fine too—it may contribute to your well-being. Overdosing on vitamins and minerals, as with anything else, may be injurious to your health.

General medical opinion—with some loud objectors and proponents of vitamin usage excepted—affirms that a good varied daily diet provides plenty of vitamins and minerals for most individuals. If you need more of certain vitamins and minerals, your physician is best qualified to advise you. If you like to spend a good part of your waking hours studying and worrying about vitamin-mineral consumption, even clocking your intake by computer, as some do, that's up to you.

246

Many people don't realize that most wholesome foods contain amounts of vitamins and minerals "naturally" (a much abused word). Chicken, for example, naturally contains not only protein and some fat, but also some calcium, iron, vitamin A, thiamin, riboflavin, and niacin.

Ask your doctor whether your last medical checkup, including blood tests and other laboratory workups, indicated any vitamin and/or mineral deficiencies for you personally.

"I understand that salads are slimming, yet I've practically lived on salads and become very heavy—how come?"

Again it's a matter of calories-IN-calories-OUT. Greens and raw vegetables are low in calories, and are a vital part of Delicious Dieting. If you add fatty meats, rich cheeses, buttery croutons, and other high-calorie ingredients, then top it all with a rich dressing, obviously you have a high-calorie, "fattening" serving.

Most salad dressings usually served in homes and restaurants amount to up to 70 or more calories per tablespoon. If you use only two tablespoons—usually more is added—you're piling on about 140 calories in salad dressing alone, equivalent to the calories in three or more heads of lettuce, more lettuce than you could eat in one salad or one sitting.

The solution when you are overweight is to eat Delicious Diet salads with D.D. dressings. You get Delicious, thoroughly satisfying taste with very few calories. That speeds you on your way to taking off excess pounds and inches rapidly, without sacrificing flavor.

Another point: You won't lose weight if you accompany your salad with heavily buttered bread or rolls—and then top off the meal with a fudge whipped-cream dessert—as we've seen many overweights do. They'll probably tell you later, "All I had was a little salad for lunch, and yet I keep gaining weight." They may fool themselves, but they can't deceive the scale.

Follow your Delicious Diet guidelines in eating salads and the other flavorful, wholesome foods on the daily menus. When you're down to your desired weight, switch to Nutri-Maintenance recommendations for preparing and eating salads and everything else. You'll stay beautifully trim, delighted by your improved good looks.

"Isn't it better to stay overweight than to lose and then regain the excess pounds?"

Absolutely not. Figure it out sensibly for yourself: To begin, there's no reason for you to regain lost weight. We can't emphasize too often that you're a person, not a statistic. Now, as never before, you have D.D. guidelines for flavorful, satisfying, low-calorie eating to help you not only slim down but stay trim lifelong. You won't gain unless you forsake the instructions. That's far less likely than in the past, since you'll be eating meals that are delicious as well as low in calories.

But let's suppose that you go down from 150 pounds to your desired weight of 124 pounds in a matter of weeks on D.D. You look and feel remarkably better and are probably much more vigorous and healthy. Then, if you personally don't care enough, let's assume that you slowly regain the 26 pounds and move up to 150 pounds over a six-month period. Realize that during that six months you averaged about 13 pounds less than when you started. Your entire system enjoyed some relief—a wonderful vacation from that 26-pound bag of groceries your body was toting around.

In the unlikely event that you put it on again, you didn't regain the 26 pounds overnight, as some dogmatic zealots would have you believe. For six months your heart and other organs were supporting up to 26 fewer pounds. That's far better than having your entire system carry the crushing weight of 150 pounds month after month. Think about it. Ask your doctor. And thumb your nose at the doomsayers who pronounce that you personally will regain lost weight because some others do. Echo Shakespeare's words: "Fie, fie on them!"

"How can overweight be considered unhealthy . . . when my obese aunt lived to 78, and I know some other very fat old people?"

Certainly a small percentage of very overweight individuals live to a ripe old age regardless of their fat. Insurance mortality tables, based on unsentimental facts, note that overweight decreases life expectancy. You must decide for yourself, based on how much you value rich overeating compared with looking and feeling your best, along with probably living longer (which nobody can guarantee).

A man I knew well was extremely overweight, a world-renowned gourmet (gourmand, we'd call him). He often patted his swollen belly proudly as he bragged, "I bet I've spent over a million dollars over the years to build this mountain. I'd rather eat and drink to the bursting point than live to a ripe old age." He died comparatively young; close friends said that he was bed-ridden in his last year.

Again—how much you weigh is your own choice. The Delicious Diet instructs you on how to slim down effectively. We're not ordering you to do so, nor are we ordering you to give up your self-esteem because you're overweight.

"Life is unfair. I have a friend who eats anything she wants and is thin as a rail. How does she get away with it?"

In the first place, your goal is to reduce yourself, not to be envious of your friend, so we hope you'll concentrate on your target unswervingly. Then you'll be so happy with your slimming results that her eating won't concern you. Beyond that, there are any number of reasons why she stays trim even though she appears to eat "anything." Most people will name "more active metabolism" as the factor, but that's just one overrated possibility.

Many such trim individuals have self-limiting eating habits. Although they appear to overeat, they stop at a certain point, limiting themselves without realizing it. Others use up many more calories by exerting more physical and nervous energy, being constantly on the go, rarely standing still—and eating only enough to satisfy themselves. Still others have eating habits that you're not aware of, such as skipping meals when you're not around.

We've questioned a number of these "eat-everything" slim people over the years and have gotten responses like these: "I dislike sweets, never eat desserts" . . . "I eat everything I want, but I loathe fatty meats and anything rich" . . . "I never have any appetite until noon, so I skip breakfast" . . . "I feel uncomfortably full if I eat between meals" . . . and on and on.

The smart thing to do is to let others eat as they wish. Their eating habits are no concern of yours. You're responsible for you, and you can become as slim as any of your trim friends—if you want to badly enough, and if you follow D.D. directions. No one ever lost an ounce through envying others and complaining that "life is unfair"—while swallowing another scoop of ice cream.

"Should I drink a lot more water than usual while on Delicious Diet?"

As you've noted in directions for the Delicious Basic Diet and the Delicious Variety Diet, no extra amounts of water are specified. For promoting general good health, drink eight glasses of water a day. It may surprise you that total water content of adults varies from 45 to 55 percent in the *obese*, to 55 to 65 percent in *thin* people.

Obviously water is necessary for life, and brings many benefits to the human system, essential in the digestive and elimination processes. Drinking enough water is also a worthy health and beauty aid for the skin. From every viewpoint, aside from being a most refreshing, calorie-free beverage, drinking plenty of water is desirable for the person in normal health. Most of us could live without food for days, weeks, and perhaps months, but not without water or substitute liquids.

"Is sleeping too much 'fattening'?"

It's questionable to label sleeping too much as "fattening," other than by noting that when you're asleep you use up fewer calories than if you're walking, exercising, or involved in active work. Certainly you shouldn't give up needed sleep as a reducing aid. Individuals vary in the hours of sleep they need to be at their best. Furthermore, just sleeping less won't make you slim—only cutting calories, as on D.D., will take off excess pounds and inches effectively.

As a matter of general interest, a British psychiatrist stated that men in their fifties who sleep nine hours a night suffer double the death rate from stroke, heart attack, or aneurysms (blood clots) than those who sleep seven hours or less. We haven't come across any authoritative corroboration of this, however.

"I think my overweight problem is due to water retention. What can I do about it?"

Water retention may be a contributing factor to being a few pounds overweight, but if you are many pounds over, it's probable that the Delicious Diet will soon bring you down to your desired weight. By all means ask your doctor to check you for a water-retention problem (which should have been noted in your last medical checkup). An increase in fiber-rich foods, and in fruits and vegetables high in vitamin C, may help keep you in balance.

In addition, your doctor will undoubtedly advise you to cut

down on your salt intake and avoid salty and smoked foods. If you're concerned about this or any medical problem, call or visit your doctor instead of worrying about a condition that may not exist.

"Shouldn't I drink a lot of whole milk on a diet, to be sure that I'm getting enough calcium?"
Milk is a fine food, but you don't need whole milk to enjoy its benefits. Skim milk is comparable nutritionally and in calcium content to whole milk but without a lot of the fat and calories. Some individuals are allergic to milk or can't tolerate it, as with some other foods. (In varied eating, as on Delicious Diets, you generally get plenty of calcium from other foods.)

"Since I'm pregnant, is it okay for me to reduce on the Delicious Diet?"
We've stated it before and it's worth stressing again: If you are pregnant, or have just had a baby, or have any illness or disorder, you should not go on any diet except one that is specified or approved by your personal physician.

"Is it better to use honey instead of sugar to cut down on calories?"
There's little difference in calories in all the sugars. Per tablespoon, granulated white sugar is 46 calories, brown sugar 52, honey 64 (surprise!), molasses 53, maple syrup 50, corn syrup 60. However, since honey is sweeter than sugar, you may use less to satisfy your taste. Sugars are simple carbohydrates that contain calories for energy only and have been called "empty calories." On the other hand, complex carbohydrates—fruits, vegetables, grains, fiber, starches—which you eat on Delicious Diets, supply energy *plus* some vitamins, minerals, and protein.

"I've substituted margarine for butter at home to cut down on calories. Isn't that much better?"
No—you don't save calories with margarine. That's a mistake many people make, no matter how often they're told. See for yourself in the calorie tables in Chapter 18. Here are the figures again per tablespoon: Butter 100 calories, margarine 100, "diet or whipped" margarine 50 to 80 calories (up to half the calories of regular margarine), vegetable oil 125, vegetable shortening 110 to 130. There are differences in consistency, and in the amounts of

251

saturated or unsaturated fat, but not in calories. Saturated fats are thick and solid at room temperature.

"Is it true, as I've read, that smoking marijuana is a help in controlling weight?"

Not from anything we've been able to learn from scientists. Marijuana contains no calories but, like alcohol and other mind-altering drugs (marijuana contains THC, which is a mind-altering drug), it can curb inhibitions about eating. It may temporarily distract you from eating—with great hunger afterward. The result can be weight gain rather than loss.

"What's the difference between creamed cottage cheese, un-creamed cottage cheese, and farmer cheese?"

There are differences in calories and texture. All are made from curdled milk drained to different degrees. Some have cream added. Calories here are for leading brands, ½ cup or 4 ounces: Creamed cottage cheese is less drained, is more moist, 115 to 120 calories. Uncreamed or low-fat cottage cheese is drained further, 90 to 100 calories. Pot cheese is drained still further, is drier, 80 to 100 calories. Farmer cheese is similar to pot cheese but is drained thoroughly, pressed, often into a bar, and is about 160 calories. But since it is denser, almost solid, one usually eats a smaller portion than with the others.

"Are foods and beverages labeled 'light' or 'lite' lower in calories than others in the same category?"

Not necessarily. At this writing there are no government standards specifying when "light" or "lite" labeling may be used or not, in relation to reduced-calorie content. Therefore some producers apply the appealing "light" labeling without reducing calories. Your only safeguard is to check and compare listings.

Watch out—"light" or "lite" on the label could be "heavy" on your body. Foods labeled "diet" or "low-calorie," however, must meet U.S. Government regulations if they are sold in interstate commerce.

"I accept the fact that calories count, but how is the caloric count in foods measured?"

All you really need to know is the calories-IN-calories-OUT equation—that if you take in more calories in foods and beverages than you expend in daily living and activity, the excess calories are stored as fat in your body, adding pounds and inches. Here's a simplified account of calorie measurement in the laboratory:

A calorie (a "large calorie" described here) is a unit of heat, the amount of heat necessary to raise the temperature of 1 kilogram of water by 1 degree centigrade. The term applies both to the heat output of an organism and to the fuel or energy value of food. The food to be measured is placed in a closed compartment called a "bomb calorimeter." It calculates the heat given off by the food in combustion (burning), and translates it into calories. Figures are checked by repeated tests, and the caloric count is established factually and dependably.

"I'm overweight and my blood pressure tends to be high. Must I really avoid highly salted and smoked foods, which I enjoy very much?"

You're foolish if you're not checked by a doctor regularly, since high blood pressure must be controlled for maximum health and long life. Overweight and high blood pressure often go together, so taking off excess weight brings some relief—but checking is still needed.

Sodium (salt) increases the retention of water in body fluids and tissues. That's highly undesirable in cases of high blood pressure, heart problems, and other health problems. Fortunately, many producers are reducing salt (sodium) content, and listing that information on labels for your guidance. Look for these salt-free or salt-reduced products now available in many types of foods.

In addition, guard against adding salt unwisely in cooking and at the table. Delicious Diets aim for lowered salt intake, but you should also be guided by your physician in order to lower your blood pressure.

"My husband has had successful heart surgery and is overweight but refuses to diet. Is it vital that he reduce?"

Here's one answer from the chief of surgery at Boston's famed Massachusetts General Hospital, where former Secretary of State Henry Kissinger had triple-bypass heart surgery for coronary heart disease. Dr. W. Gerald Austen said that Kissinger, his considerably overweight patient, had lost ten pounds in the hospital and needed to lose twenty more. Dr. Austen stated flatly, "The most important thing, and all kidding aside, is that he should lose that weight."

"Is yogurt really a miracle food for reducing and staying slim?"

No, there are no "miracle foods," no matter what partisans may claim about yogurt or anything else. Yogurt is good, nutritious food—period. It's relatively low in calories in relation to bulk food content, but far from being calorie free. Low-fat yogurt per cup is about 110 to 150 calories . . . plain whole-milk yogurt is 140 to 160 (comparable to milk), fruited yogurt up to 270 calories (largely because of added sugar). Check calorie listings on containers.

The highly touted longevity factor claimed for yogurt hasn't been proved scientifically. While yogurt provides desirable amounts of calcium, protein, carbohydrates, some vitamins and minerals, it's fairly high in sodium generally—as is milk. Yogurt brings you many benefits, but a cupful won't turn you into Wonder Woman or Superman, nor slim you automatically despite what any advertiser may imply.

Millions of overweight women and men would like simply to swallow a magic pill, and lo! slim, trim, and twenty years younger forever. It won't work, any more than swallowing a magic pill will make you rich. And now, back to what *does* work. . . .

"My parents and their parents were fat, so overweight runs in my family. Am I therefore destined to be overweight always, as I am now?"

Overweight doesn't necessarily run in families, but overeating high-calorie foods often does—usually excessively fatty foods and rich desserts in oversize portions. Your first step is a medical checkup. If your doctor assures you that your metabolism, thyroid, and other bodily processes are functioning normally, there's no physical reason why you can't achieve the slimness you want.

Just follow the Delicious Quick-Trim Diet exactly. You'll very quickly stop being concerned about "family overweight" as you lose weight swiftly and permanently.

"I'm happily passing up high-calorie desserts and other favorite foods because I'm slimming down so beautifully on D.D. Will I ever be able to indulge?"

You certainly will—as soon as you're down to your desired weight. Then you can follow D.D. Nutri-Maintenance Eating guidelines and indulge in some foods you think you miss. (Don't be surprised if you can't stand some of those former favorites because they're too rich and fatty for your improved taste.) As directed, you'll settle on your own calories-IN-calories-OUT equation to stay trim.

"I've lost fifteen pounds in two weeks on D.D., and I'm thrilled about it—but a fat, envious neighbor says that it's all 'water loss.' Is she right?"

Show your envious neighbor Chapter 4, "The Scientific How"—especially the explanation about losing "only water." She'll learn that on D.D. one loses both fat and water as fat cells are thrown off—and that *the water is not regained unless the fat is regained.* Perhaps she'll be so impressed that she'll go on the Delicious Diet and become sylphlike herself, her envy replaced by joy in her newly slim figure.

"Does the Delicious Diet reduce 'cellulite'?"

You probably ask that question because some self-professed reducing specialists, particularly in the exercise area, have made big promises about reducing "cellulite." They refer to it as a unique kind of fat that vanishes with their special reducing methods. Medical experts give this little or no credence.

Discussing this in a public forum, an informed physician said that he'd never come across "cellulite" in his research: "I do know that fat is fat is fat—and too much fat and too many calories in the diet will make you fat." To sum up then: If you take in fewer calories than you use up daily, you'll get rid of fat, whatever it's labeled. By any name, your Delicious Diet will trim it off and keep you slim.

"If I'm allergic to any of the foods on the Delicious Diet, do I have to eat them anyhow?"

Absolutely not. Substitute any of the delicious, nutritious comparable foods on D.D., as stated in the detailed directions. As you'll note, personal choice is an integral part of reducing pleasantly the *Delicious* way.

"Can I have 'coffee breaks' on D.D.?"

Yes, whenever it's most convenient for you personally. Just stay within D.D. regulations for snacks and beverages.

"I'm delighted at the prospect of losing up to a pound or more a day with Delicious Dieting, but won't losing weight so fast make me weak?"

No, quite the opposite is true. You'll be relieving your body from the burden of excess pounds that had to be supported by your heart, legs, feet, back—indeed, your entire system. You'll be thrilled by how much lighter and more active you feel as well as by how much more attractive you look. Just think—carrying around a heavy package all day is what weakens you, not putting it down.

> *"Like any sensible person, I know what moderate portions are, of course, but when I'm permitted steak on D.D., for example, I'm capable of eating a two-pound steak. What do I do about that?"*

Simply ask yourself, "Do I want to slim down—or do I want to prove how much I can eat?" If your answer is the latter, then you won't lose weight on D.D. or any other diet. If you truly want to slim down, observe the guidelines precisely, and you'll soon achieve the trim, more vigorous, healthier body that's your goal. Remember to trim all fat and to chew your steak portion (three to four ounces) slowly. You will enjoy the flavor to the fullest—and indeed feel full.

> *"I went to a wedding, stuffed myself, breaking my diet, of course, and was sick that night—but what else could I do on such a joyous occasion?"*

You could and should have eaten moderately of the foods available within D.D. guidelines. There is a wide choice you can enjoy, as you know. Plus, you could have merely relaxed the rules somewhat, as discussed before, sipped a whiskey and soda, a dry martini, or a glass of dry Champagne.

Then you could have made up for the special eating by going on the One-Day Liquid Diet the next day, or simply returning to your regular Delicious Diet—and started losing weight rapidly again, with no guilt feelings.

Above all, as warned before, *don't ever overstuff yourself.* Overloading at any one meal can trigger physical breakdowns, heart attacks, and other ills—just as overloading a truck can cause it to break down.

> *"If I get a cold while dieting, shouldn't I eat more, since they say that one should 'feed a cold'?"*

No, that's an outmoded, erroneous concept. If you get a cold, fever, or other illness when overweight, stuffing yourself only makes you more uncomfortable, not better. If you're concerned about your cold, don't hesitate to call your doctor, describe your symptoms, temperature, and so on, and abide by his instructions.

"Does slimming down usually improve sexual performance?"
There are too many physical, emotional, and psychological influences bearing on sexual potency to credit or blame slimness or overweight one way or another. Some partners may be turned off by excess fat and flab. In other cases, obesity may interfere with physical comfort and general vigor. But no one can make any valid promise that slimming down increases sexual desire or potency. Sorry. But that doesn't mean it may not happen!

"Is it desirable to eat 'health foods' on D.D.?"
That's up to you—it's not necessary at all. You can buy so-called health foods if you prefer, always within D.D. guidelines, but they're generally more expensive and not necessarily more nutritious. Just because something is labeled "health food" or bought in a "health food store" doesn't automatically make it healthier. Furthermore, check labels for calories, fat, and other undesirable elements before you buy, since a "health food" isn't specifically low calorie.

Along the same lines, don't be misled by the word *"natural"* on a label. "Natural" is not necessarily better or more healthful. Poisonous plants, for example, are "natural" but not safe and certainly not healthful. Look for desirable specifics, such as "no salt added," or "no sugar added." Remind yourself of the *New Yorker* cartoon that shows a man in a coffee shop asserting, "I won't eat anything but natural foods, like meat and potatoes."

"Are the calorie differences in foods labeled 'low calorie' important in losing weight?"
The differences can be considerable in lowering your calorie intake, but you must check the contents labels to be sure. Some brands of bottled Russian dressing reveal as many as 90 calories per tablespoon; a "low-calorie" brand may have as few as 4 calories—a significant saving. Tasteful D.D. dressing recipes always cut your calorie intake with luscious flavor.

Unfortunately, some local producers label products "lower in calories" or "lowered calories" without really reducing calories much. The phrases are intended to lure calorie-conscious shoppers, but you won't be deceived if you check the calories on comparable brands.

"I read that fat babies—I was one—develop 'fat cells' that keep them overweight for life. Does that mean I'll never be slim, no matter what I do?"

There's much confusion about "fat cells," but one thing is positive—that multitudes of individuals (including me, once a fat baby) are now slim, trim, active adults. "Fat cells" are used as an excuse by many people for overeating and being under-active. If you're in normal health, go on the Delicious Quick-Trim Diet, stick with it, and you can't help but slim down, regardless of concern about "fat cells."

"Friends tell me that hot tubs, saunas, and heat cabinets are a sure way to take off excess pounds. Is that true?"

Many people enjoy sitting in hot tubs, saunas, and the like, and some become overly enthusiastic about the health-building and reducing effects. Enjoy these heat treatments if you like— and if they don't exhaust you—but you're not likely to slim down unless you eat fewer calories than you expend. Incidentally, have you ever noticed that many devotees of hot tubs, saunas, and steam baths are overweight and even obese?

"Should I take massage and vibrator treatments to lose weight?"

If massages and the use of vibrating devices and machines make you feel good and don't harm you—enjoy. But don't expect them to reduce you, regardless of claims. As one dermatologist explained, "Basically, massaging and vibrating just push your skin around—on your body or face—and loosen the skin, which is hardly desirable."

Many of the answers to the questions here, as noted at the start, have appeared at various points in this book. If questions come up as you proceed with Delicious Dieting, please read the D.D. Guidelines carefully again. This is your slim-down and stay-trim "bible." Referring to it as needed can assure you a trim, most attractive body for the rest of your potentially healthier, more active, longer life.

Concluding this section is probably the most-asked question of all:

"I'm afraid to face another letdown since I've failed on so many diets before—or perhaps they've failed me. How can I have faith that Delicious Dieting will work for me?"

Because you've never been on a diet before that is so high in gratifying taste and eating enjoyment, and still low in calories. The proof is in trying the Delicious Quick-Trim Diet of your choice for just one week. Then see the wonderful slimming-trimming difference for yourself on the scale and in the full-length mirror. By following directions exactly you can't miss—*success at last!*

20

Bonus Pointers for Quick-Trim Success and _____Lifelong Slimness

Here are some tips, comments, and recommendations, a number of them based on letters or remarks from dieters. Some of the pointers have been touched on before, but they deserve to be repeated from a different angle. They should be as helpful to you as they have been to others.

GIVE YOURSELF A BREAK . . .

"When I'm tempted to take a midmorning coffee break at home," Marion S. advises, "I often take an activity break instead. I turn on the TV and enjoy walking briskly or jogging in place in front of the set. I get my blood flowing and work up a mild sweat while watching a tearful soap opera. It cheers me up to know I'm getting rid of calories instead of adding them, and I return to my work invigorated rather than bloated."

We commend Marion S. and suggest that she can enjoy a hardly-any-calories coffee break, if she pleases, after her activity break with a cup of coffee or tea and a satisfying *D.D. Fudgy Chocolate Meringue, only 30 calories.

WHEN IS "NUTRITIOUS" NUTRITIOUS?

Here's another example of the necessity for reading the fine print on food packages, not just the advertised promises:

260

Combination cranberry-apple juice is a refreshing, tasty drink. One brand advertises in large print that "tangy cranberries plus juicy apples equal clean, crisp refreshment." True—and it sounds nutritious. Let's check the small print on the package:

Ingredients are listed in order of their predominance: "filtered water, cranberry juice, high-fructose corn syrup, apple juice from concentrate, natural apple flavor, fumaric acid, and vitamin C." Fine—now you know that the product contains more water than either cranberry juice or apple juice, and more high-fructose corn syrup—that's sugar—than apple juice. Being informed, you can compare fruit juices and make your buying decision intelligently—and nutritiously.

Comparing *calories* in a 6-ounce glass: cranberry-apple juice 130 calories; these no-sugar-added juices—apple juice 80 calories, grapefruit juice 70, orange juice 80 calories. That specifies the slim-trim difference for you.

"I DRESS UP D.D. DISHES . . ."

Diana W. advises, "I've noticed that when most people I know go on a reducing diet, their attitude generally is that the food will be tasteless and unsatisfying, so they're going to sacrifice and suffer. Therefore they tend to dish out the food without attention or care, as though it's slop. With such a defeatist approach, no wonder so many dieters fail. On the other hand, I expected to find Sylvia Schur's D.D. recipes perfectly delicious—and they are.

"I go a step further in serving them—I arrange a salad decoratively on a bed of varied greens . . . sometimes sprinkle on a little shredded coconut and perhaps some grated ginger . . . a few almond slivers or chopped nuts on stuffed tomatoes, for example . . . chopped chives on soup served in our loveliest bowls . . . sesame, caraway, or poppy seeds, sometimes combinations, on chicken or fish . . . arranging the D.D. vegetables colorfully on my best guest platter.

"I get a creative kick out of planning and carrying through these attractive touches. My family and guests appreciate the tempting appearance, as I do—and we all enjoy the delectable servings immensely, not even thinking or knowing that they're low in calories. One expects fine gourmet recipes to be served beautifully—and that's exactly what Delicious Diet dishes are."

261

GOING BANANAS . . .

"As a perfectly Delicious Diet dessert—or for enjoying any time," Natalie B. writes, "I recommend freezing a banana. Couldn't be simpler to prepare: Peel a banana. Cut it in half if you wish, and insert a wooden pop stick in each half. Sprinkle with lemon juice, and cover it tightly with plastic wrap. Freeze until ready to eat as a frozen treat, either as a frozen pop, or with a spoon.

"For another variation, mash the peeled ripe banana, sprinkle and mix in some lemon juice and place in a small freezer container. Cover and keep in the freezer. Before eating, take out and let thaw for a few minutes, then dig in with a spoon. It tastes like a luscious banana sundae—but it's just sweet natural banana, with no added calories."

SOME UN-SALTY SUGGESTIONS . . .

Medical science warns increasingly that while a little salt is essential for humans, too much salt can be unhealthy. Normally the body needs less than one-tenth of a teaspoon of salt per day— but most people consume two to three teaspoons of salt, over twenty times the amount required. Most doctors agree that salt may promote high blood pressure and accelerate the risks of stroke and heart attack.

If you think we're all born with a need for lots of salt in our daily eating, you're mistaken. Much salt is not required by the human system, it's an *acquired* taste. It has been shown that children fed from early years without salt did well in eating and enjoying their food; they didn't find it "tasteless," as some salt-conditioned adults would claim.

You should reduce your salt intake, especially if your doctor advised that you cut down at your last visit. Here are some simple aids to consider:

- When shopping, take the time to check for the salt content in foods—increasingly being listed on labels. Take advantage of the great variety of products, more each year, labeled "no salt added," "low sodium," and "reduced sodium." Salt, remember, is about 40 percent sodium.
  As for availability, at this writing, *The New York Times*

262

reported, "Two large producers of canned goods announced plans to market vegetables without salt." One company, the world's largest fruit and vegetable canner, was introducing a new no-salt-added line of green beans, corn, tomato sauce and paste, and peas. Another company was converting one of its leading lines of canned vegetables to no-salt, no-sugar-added products, including peas, corn, lima beans, mushrooms, carrots, and spinach. Some are available now.

- Be assured on D.D., and in general everyday eating, that if you have no abnormality you get plenty of sodium from the vegetables, poultry, fish, meat, and other foods you eat. So, even when we perspire, we need not be concerned about getting too little sodium.
- A little salt used in cooking usually isn't harmful, except in severe cases of high blood pressure and heart conditions, which should be under a doctor's close supervision. There's no point in becoming fanatical about cutting down on salt, but one obvious move is to keep the salt shaker off the dining table, removing that temptation from habitual salt overusers, who tend to use it without thinking.
- Try seasoning with your favorite herbs and spices instead of salt. Those that are sodium-free include allspice, anise, basil, bay leaf, caraway, cayenne, chervil, chili powder, cinnamon, cloves, curry powder, dill, fennel, garlic, ginger, juniper, mace, marjoram, mint, dry mustard, nutmeg, oregano, paprika, pepper, pimiento, rosemary, sage, savory, tarragon, thyme. Stores have salt-free mixtures now.
- Don't be misled by packages labeled "herb seasoning," or "all-purpose herb/spice seasoning"—these seasonings are not necessarily salt-free. Check contents on labels.
- "Iodized" salt (treated with iodine or an iodide) is recommended, since a very small amount of the chemical iodine is generally needed by humans. It's possible, however, that enough of the chemical is in other foods that you eat.

EASY DOES IT . . .

Gulping your food, hardly chewing at all, tends to leave your appetite unsatisfied, since you've hardly tasted anything at all. Keep reminding yourself to chew s-l-o-w-l-y, to take your time in order to enjoy every bit thoroughly. Be aware of what you are eating and tasting. If you bolt down your food and drink, you'll find yourself looking at an empty plate or glass barely conscious of what you've swallowed.

You'll find that you'll get more flavor gratification from each calorie you consume—and that fewer calories provide more satisfaction. There are many simple and Delicious ways of s-t-r-e-t-c-h-i-n-g out the food you eat.

For example, instead of finishing off an apple in a few huge bites, core and cut it into about eight segments (an inexpensive apple corer will core an apple and divide it into appealing segments in one simple motion). Eat and chew the segments slowly for greater enjoyment.

Invent other stretchers, too—such as cutting up a banana into thin, round slices and eating each individually, instead of making the luscious fruit disappear in a few bites. Also, try arranging the separate segments of an orange attractively on a plate before eating.

VERMOUTH VARIATION . . .

"You hear a lot about cooking with wine," says a fine amateur cook, Dan K., "but I find that in many cases using a little dry vermouth adds a special tangy flavor. I've had Delicious results with vermouth in an herb marinade, which I use in broiling, and in a lightly seasoned salad dressing. After all, vermouth is just a wine in which herbs have been steeped in various combinations."

CLUCKING OVER CHICKEN DOGS . . .

If you and your family go for hot dogs, you might try "chicken dogs" instead of the beef or meat frankfurters. A chicken frank averages about 120 calories—while meat frankfurters usually run 150 calories or more for the same size sausage. Some packages of chicken dogs are marked "sodium-reduced." Low-sodium mustard is also available. And chicken bologna and other pressed-meat products are being offered in many stores.

DON'T BE FOOLED BY COSTLY WORDS . . .

Beware of food producers who raise their prices when they put words such as "diet," "low calorie," or "reduced calories" on products without changing any of the ingredients. As one specific example, Judy N. says, "In the diet food section of a large supermarket I found a brand of 'diet sardines' that was priced at 89¢. Checking the regular shelves of sardines, I came upon the same brand, with the same ingredients and the same number of calories.

"The difference was that the word 'diet' was eliminated from the label—and the item was sold at 85¢, five percent less. No way could it cost four cents more per can to print 'diet' on the label. I've found many instances where it pays in actual savings to read labels, and compare contents, listings, and costs."

A GENTLE, SPARKLING TOUCH . . .

"Guests love it when I serve my special fruit cup as dessert," says Peggy H., "yet there's nothing magical about it, merely a gentle, sparkling touch of liqueur added at the last minute—along with a few fresh mint leaves on top. It doesn't matter which liqueur I use, just a few drops of whatever is handy and open.

"If we're serving Champagne or a dry sparkling wine, I add a bit of that instead of liqueur. The result isn't just an ordinary dish of cut-up fruit, but a specially pleasing D.D. dessert treat." A word of caution—when you pour, make sure to use only a touch of liqueur lest you add too many extra calories.

DRIPPY REMINDER . . .

When broiling or baking poultry or meat, don't forget to place it on a rack high enough for the fat to drip off into a pan below. This will eliminate a greasy taste and texture, too.

BREAKING THE SUGAR HABIT . . .

"A big help to me in staying trim," says Mary T., "since I drink a lot of tea and coffee through the day, is keeping the number 18 prominently in mind. That's the number of calories in each teaspoon of sugar, of course. I drink at least six cups a day and used to stir in two teaspoons of sugar per cup. When I discovered that I was adding over 200 calories a day in sugar alone, I omitted sweetening entirely, and now find that I enjoy the true coffee and tea flavors much more."

Of course you may use noncaloric sugar substitutes if you prefer; you'll get plenty of energy from the carbohydrates in fruits, vegetables, and other foods in Delicious Dieting and in D.D. Nutri-Maintenance Eating.

PRE-WRAP SNACK PACKS . . .

An excellent way to snack and satisfy your taste without adding lots of calories is to pre-wrap snacks. Place the nibbles in a container in the refrigerator so you can reach in and help yourself as you wish. And accomplish the same with an airtight pre-wrap to take to work. Pack marinated carrot strips and raw zucchini slices, raw or marinated mushrooms, cucumber spears, fresh fruit such as grapes and cherries, or any of the other low-calorie Delicious Diet edibles described in this book.

SCISSORING OFF CALORIES . . .

Laura V. has found that "you can cut off more fat from raw and cold cooked meat with a sharp scissors than you can with the sharpest knife. I keep a special 'food scissors' handy among the cooking knives for just such extra calorie-cutting purposes."

DRY UP CALORIES . . .

"Dry" in wine means less sugar, so you're cutting calories when you drink a dry rather than sweet wine. The dry wine may seem a bit too tart at first, but when you become accustomed to that crisp, clean taste, you'll wonder how you ever tolerated wines that some call "cloyingly sweet." A 4-ounce glass of dry white or red wine contains about 85 calories on average, whereas the sweet wine can total up to 200 calories—more than double the calories.

When ordering broiled fish in a restaurant remember to specify "broiled dry." (At home, of course, you can use a tasteful D.D. wine marinade.) Done correctly, the fish will arrive at the table moist and tender, without the calories of butter, oil, or margarine used in broiling by many chefs.

PLEASING YOUR HOSTESS . . .

"I use a little forgivable subterfuge," says Eleanor H., "when hors d'oeuvres are served before dinner. I take one small appetizer, nibble it slowly and enjoy it thoroughly—but I pass up all the rest, no matter how many times offered to me. I tell my hostess how absolutely marvelous the delicacy was that I ate—she is pleased and I haven't loaded in a *lot* of calories."

FILLING UP ON NO-CALORIE BEVERAGES . . .

Many dieters advise that it helps them to fill up before and during meals with hot or iced decaffeinated coffee, hot or iced tea, club soda, no-sugar sodas, and water. They get a feeling of fullness that helps formerly big eaters from loading up with high-calorie food. Of course, eating the D.D. way prevents consuming excess calories—but you may find the extra no-calorie drinking an aid. Water has been called a "vital nutrient" for internal cleansing and flushing out the system.

You'll run into some people who say that drinking so much liquid makes them feel bloated. What really makes one feel "over-beveraged" is being "oversalted" from taking in too much salt in foods, and even in high-sodium soups, club soda, and "naturally carbonated" waters. Buy salt-free seltzer or soda instead. If you overload with sodium bicarbonate and other salt-containing antacids, you may be oversalting your system again. Most of us need not be extreme about it, but it's wise to check labels for sodium content. To avoid excess *sweetness*, mix diet soda and seltzer, half and half.

"DON'T BE A SWEET ROLL SNATCHER . . ."

"If I had one tip for others who have reduced beautifully on D.D., as I have," says Alice S., "it would be to clamp down on sweet rolls and other breads in restaurants and at home. I'm tempted particularly when there are sweet rolls such as blueberry muffins and honeybuns present. I was shocked to learn that even a hard roll thickly buttered adds up to 300 calories.

"My own lifelong Nutri-Maintenance plan is to select very carefully the one roll or slice of bread I like best, eat it bit by bit without added butter, or with the slightest touch of butter or jam—and that's all. To make up for that indulgence, I cut down on what I eat during the rest of the meal. Thus I cater to my personal preferences, and stay slim."

STAYING TRIM "ON THE SIDE" . . .

You can actually save hundreds of calories, and keep pounds from piling on, by taking salad dressings "on the side" at home and in restaurants. Even when serving the family at home, you can mix the salad with dressing for the others, but leave a plain portion for yourself—then add dressing to suit and slim yourself.

At home, use flavorful low-calorie D.D. dressing recipes, low-calorie bottled dressings, or fresh lemon juice or vinegar. In restaurants, ask for fresh lemon juice and available seasonings. More and more restaurants offer a variety of seasonings available so patrons can mix dressings to their personal taste.

Don't be self-conscious about asking. For years, self-confident gourmets have insisted on mixing their own dressings in fine restaurants. Some individuals even carry a packet of their own seasonings.

Even if the restaurant serves only rich dressings, when you order "dressing on the side," you are in control. If you wish to indulge some, you can add just a touch of the dressing—instead of having the kitchen staff load hundreds—yes, hundreds—of extra calories on your salad.

"SKIP THE HARD CANDY SNACK . . ."

A formerly overweight Delicious dieter said that "a heavy woman in our office came up with the idea of having a bowl of hard candies around for snacking. She claimed that eating one hard candy would satisfy hunger and keep down appetites. The others approved, in spite of my being against it.

"I said it might work if each could stop at one hard candy for the day, but such restraint wasn't likely. I kept count and found that the fattest women and men there had their fingers in the candy bowl all day. They were consuming hundreds of *extra* sugar calories on the pretext of curbing their appetites. The boss decided wisely that out of sight and out of reach meant out of overloaded stomachs."

VEGETABLE LIST PROVIDES LATITUDE . . .

When Dorothy G. told friends that vegetables were a vital part of her Delicious Diet, they claimed that the selection of vegetables available was just too limiting. She explains, "I made up a list of vegetables that are 50 calories or less for a generous full-cup serving, or a comparable measure." Her friends were impressed by the great variety. Here's her list:

VEGETABLES . . . CALORIES PER CUP OR COMPARABLE SERVING

	calories		calories
Asparagus (6 spears)	20	Kale	45
Bean sprouts (raw)	26	Lettuce (loose leaf head)	30
Beans, green	25	Mushrooms	41
Beans, wax	22	Okra (cooked)	30
Broccoli	50	Onion (raw)	50
Brussels sprouts	50	Peppers, sweet (medium)	20
Cabbage (cooked)	40	Radishes (6 small)	15
Cabbage (raw)	25	Sauerkraut	30
Carrots (raw)	20	Spinach	45
Cauliflower	30	Squash, summer	35
Celery	20	Tomatoes (cooked)	45
Chard, Swiss	30	Turnips	40
Cucumber (raw)	16	Watercress	10
Eggplant	34	Zucchini	35
Endive	10		

STICK TO NO-STICK . . .

Get out of the habit of using the skillet every time you fry or sauté food. Automatically you're tossing in hundreds of extra calories before cooking by greasing the pan with butter, oil, margarine, or other fats. Instead use a no-stick pan, add a little low-sodium broth, or a few squirts of vegetable cooking spray—practically no calories. You might even use a touch of sweet butter instead, but on the whole it's best to avoid the added fats.

"TV CAN BE DANGEROUS TO YOUR HEALTH . . ."

"That's true," a loving wife told us. "I finally got my very over-weight husband to go on the Delicious Diet, thanks to his doctor's emphatic orders after a severe heart attack. John was losing weight, but not fast enough, and I was puzzled. Then, when I returned from shopping one Saturday, I came upon him watching a ball-game on TV, loading himself with potato chips and beer.

"I substituted a bowl of D.D. snacks and a can of no-sugar soda, and he admitted that he was so intent on the game he'd hardly noticed the switch. He granted that it was the *act of eating* that he was used to, and he was satisfied as long as he was nibbling and drinking. I keep plenty of the low-calorie items around, and he's been taking off the excess pounds ever since."

BECOME A D.D. DUO . . .

A good many beautifully slimmed couples have told us that they found it particularly satisfying to trim down as a D.D. duo—turning their daily weight loss into a sort of contest. You might consider trying this as couples, with friends, neighbors, even relatives who live far away. Check each other's weights and di-mensions in person, or by phone, or letter. D.D. is the basis for a healthy, happy "reducing game," leading to lifelong rewards.

ENJOY A "D.D. AQUA-COOLER" INSTEAD OF WATER . . .

A creative friend, Jane S., who slimmed down beautifully on the Delicious Basic Diet, says that her favorite no-calorie drink while dieting and since is one she invented herself, a D.D. Aqua-Cooler:

"I use a tall, slim glass with a frosted finish, fill it with bottled spring water and crushed ice, then top it with a bit of colorful fruit—a couple of fresh raspberries or a thin-sliced strawberry, sliver of banana, kiwi, lemon or orange, a pitted cherry, a couple of halved grapes, even grapefruit—whatever is handy.

"That touch of color from the fruit, topped with a sprig of mint or watercress, makes it look like a party drink. It's refreshing, healthful—and look, Ma, no calories!"

EGG-LOVER'S POINTER . . .

"I love eggs," Corinne T. reports, "but I limit myself because of the cholesterol content. What I do is eat only the whites, which are cholesterol-free. They're not as flavorful as whole eggs, but I find that it satisfies my yen when I scramble them with a little skim milk, cut-up bits of tomato, green pepper, onion, parsley, chives—whatever I have handy—plus a touch of grated Romano cheese and herbs. If you'll pardon the expression, it makes an eggs-citing dish."

POP POPCORN INTO YOUR MOUTH?

Be wary of any diet advice that recommends popcorn as a frequent low-calorie snack. Popcorn is literally popped corn—and corn itself is far from low in calories. For the benefit of your slimmed figure, here are figures to keep in mind.

Plain popcorn (with no salt or butter) contains about 30 calories per cup. Add a little butter, salt, cheese or cheese flavor, and you're up to 200 calories or more per cup. Reach for caramel-coated popcorn, and you'll be consuming up to 300 calories per cup.

The clear lesson is to pop popcorn in your mouth only if you pop it plain. Once down to your desired weight, you can indulge according to D.D. Nutri-Maintenance guidelines.

PUTTING THE FREEZE ON CALORIES . . .

"I use a lot of frozen vegetables," says Nancy P., "since I spend a long day in the office and have little time to shop and cook. Last night I was shocked when I compared packages of frozen mixed vegetables in my freezer. . . .

271

"Plain mixed vegetables had 58 calories per half-cup. The same vegetables in butter sauce (which doesn't taste very buttery) had 83 calories. A half cup of mixed vegetables with onion sauce contained 120 calories—more than double the calories of plain. From now on it's plain frozen vegetables for me!"

"MIXTURES ADD TEXTURES FOR MORE FLAVOR . . ."

"I've invented ways to take advantage of food textures to add to the taste and eye appeal of D.D. dishes," says Helen P., "and I enjoy what I eat even more. When I'm having my dry cereal at D.D. Wednesday breakfast, I use a pre-prepared no-sugar-added mixture of my own. In a large, airtight glass jar, I keep a mixture of whole wheat flakes, oats, bran, puffed rice, and wheat mini-biscuits. I pour the mix into a bowl and enjoy it much more than one type of cereal alone.

"When I scramble eggs for the family and myself at D.D. Sunday breakfast, I whip in some chopped pimiento, grated onion or chopped chives, bits of asparagus or other leftover vegetables that add flavor and color. I heat the mixture slowly in a no-stick pan, and serve it on lovely floral-design dishes. Everyone raves about this D.D. treat, which is so much tastier and more satisfying than plain scrambled eggs."

BE AWARE OF DIFFERING CALORIES IN BREAD . . .

When you're having a slice of bread or toast while on your Delicious Diet, or during Nutri-Maintenance Eating, bear in mind that some breads have more calories than others—and the differences can be significant. No, you don't count calories on D.D., but there are helpful lessons in the calorie charts and the information on labels. Here are just a few instances of the surprising range of differences:

	calories		*calories*
Thin-slice white bread	40	*Whole-wheat*	*50–80*
Regular white bread	*60–80*	*Date-nut*	90
Protein	45	*Dense pumpernickel*	100
Gluten	50	*Oatmeal-raisin*	120
High-fiber bran	90		

Note that the bread with the highest calorie content has *triple* the calories of the lowest. Such comparisons, of breads as well as other types of food, can certainly help you slim down and stay trim forever.

Here are some recommendations that appear elsewhere in this book but that bear repetition:

- When table d'hote or full-course meals are listed prominently on a menu, don't just order them automatically. Look instead for the à la carte offerings—if you don't see them, ask the waiter. You'll avoid the pressure of stuffing a full-course meal into yourself—and groaning when you step on the scale next morning.
- Always order salad dressing "on the side," making a specific point of this without fail. That way you can apply a spoonful or two of your favorite dressing instead of a large amount— already mixed in and beyond your control. Furthermore, greens often go limp when overdressed, or when the sauce is mixed in long before the salad is served.
- Order your fish broiled "dry"; that is, cooked with a little wine and/or lemon juice instead of butter, margarine, or oil.
- Ask whether the entrée is served with a rich, heavy sauce or gravy. If so, tell the waiter to leave it off, or to serve it on the side. If you're told it can't be done with this dish, order something else.
- When you specify "prepared dry" or "without sauce or gravy," and the food is served otherwise—don't hesitate to send it back. Be gracious but firm. There's no reason for you to add unwanted fat and extra calories because the waiter or chef made a mistake.
- In a Chinese restaurant, remember that fried rice has three times the calories of steamed rice. If you've allowed for these extra calories (or some other dish in any restaurant), *enjoy*— you've planned it that way.
- If your "lean hamburger" arrives served with potato chips or French fries, remember that every chip adds about 20 calories, and that French fries add even more, plus lots of extra salt and fat. Guide your eating accordingly. If you had asked, you might have been able to get a little lettuce and sliced tomato instead. Think about it beforehand.

273

- Keep in mind that if you specify extra lemon wedges with your fish, salads, or other servings, you'll be adding lots of sparkling flavor—and no calories.
- In most restaurants, appetizers such as a cold half-lobster may be ordered as your entrée instead—a worthwhile choice if you wish to save calories, and money.
- Even if *broiled* poultry, fish, and meats aren't listed on a menu, you can usually get them broiled "without added fats," if you ask.
- If you're ordering alcoholic drinks, remember that "dry" means not only less sweet but also lower in calories. That's true of dry wines; and order whiskey with water or club soda (preferably salt-free seltzer) instead of ginger ale, or a dry martini instead of a sweet manhattan. For an after-dinner drink, dry Cognac or brandy is preferable to a sweet cordial (1 ounce of dry brandy has about 60 calories, as compared to 100 or more for a sweet cordial).
- If you're feeling pleasantly satisfied, and there is still food left on your plate (such as a chicken leg, some steak, and so on), don't try to finish it. Instead, ask that it be wrapped for you to take along—that's done acceptably now in the finest eating places.

Our favorite maître d' in one of the country's top restaurants told us, "Our self-assured patrons don't hesitate to ask to take home uneaten food—it would be silly for them not to, since they've paid for it. Our chef considers take-home a compliment to his cooking."

REDUCING YOUR CALORIES-FAT-SALT INTAKE . . .

While on your Delicious Diet, you've found out happily that you lose up to a pound or more a day deliciously, simply by carefully following directions. When you switch to D.D. Nutri-Maintenance Eating, guided by your scale and the many recommendations in this book, you can benefit by selecting the foods that are lower in fat, salt, and calories. Here are some tips to head you in the right direction:

- Reduced-calorie mayonnaise has less than half the calories of regular mayonnaise and about half the cholesterol.
- Lighter maple-flavored syrups have about one-third the cal-

ories of regular maple syrup (there's a difference in flavor, of course).

- You can get "diet" salad dressings with as few as 5 calories per tablespoon, as compared to 100 calories per tablespoon for other bottled dressings. Certainly there's a difference in flavor, but judging by sales, many people find the "diet" salad dressings satisfactory. And some report that they can't tell the difference when eating a flavorful, varied salad.

  Your best bet is to use low-calorie D.D. salad dressing recipes—truly gratifying. It's easy to mix some in a bottle, and keep in the refrigerator for future use.

- Fruit spreads—jams, jellies, preserves—are available with as few as 6 calories per tablespoon, compared with up to 60 calories (ten times as many) in regular packaged varieties. Whatever you choose, save calories by spreading the jam thin rather than piling it on thickly. Try D.D. fruit spread recipes, which cut down on calories but never on luscious, satisfying flavor.

- Cheeses range from standard types such as American and Swiss at 105 to 115 calories per ounce, 8 to 10 grams of fat, and 25 to 30 milligrams of cholesterol; down to "reduced-calorie" cheese with 50 calories per ounce, 2 grams of fat, and 10 milligrams of cholesterol. Quite a difference in calories—and admittedly quite a contrast in flavor and texture. Decide for yourself.

  New "lighter" products are coming on the market each month, and many—such as the tasty varieties of low-calorie crackers and flatbreads, are worth sampling.

"I DON'T COOK 'DIET FOOD,' I SERVE D.D."

One of the most pleasing compliments we've received, and we've heard it from many people, parallels this enthusiastic comment from Marjorie T. "Our family has enjoyed D.D. recipes so much that this has become my regular way of cooking for guests, too.

"The praise has been wonderful for my ego. At times when I've told guests after a meal that they've been eating low-calorie D.D. dishes, they've expressed special delight that they ate so deliciously without eating high calorie. I don't consider your recipes as diet foods, but rather as a most desirable and healthful way of eating."

275

21

Longer Life the D.D. Quick-Trim and Nutri-Maintenance Way

Strong medical opinion confirms the evidence that being slim and trim increases your chances for good health and longer life—and that being overweight does damage to your system, not just externally in bulging inches, but also internally as well.

Our combined experience has taught us that being at one's desired weight is more likely to lead to *happier* living than being weighed down by excess pounds. We consider that true for almost everyone, in spite of the many variables that add up to "happiness." You *don't* need the added burden of oppressive weight as another of life's complications. No one can guarantee you longer life and happiness. You can be slim and seemingly in "perfect health," yet be brought down by severe illness or unrelated accident. It has been said that "fate laughs at probabilities," but you should be determined to do your best to shape your body and destiny for your most rewarding and enduring life.

Inside practically every ballooning, overweight, and overburdened body is a potentially trimmer, healthier, happier person. If you are overweight and happy, blessings on you—this book was not written for you; it's for those who want to be trim and attractive—and to accomplish it *Deliciously*.

For your further benefit, let's look at some other important factors affecting slimness, optimum health, and longer life.

EFFECT OF FAT ON CANCER

A report released in 1982 by the prestigious Committee on Diet, Nutrition, and Cancer of the National Research Council is summed up in this brief excerpt:

> In general, the evidence suggests that some types of diets and some dietary components (e.g., high-fat diets or the frequent consumption of salt-cured, salt-pickled, and smoked foods) tend to increase the risk of cancer, whereas others (e.g., low-fat diets or the frequent consumption of certain fruits and vegetables) tend to decrease it.

The Delicious Quick-Trim Basic Diet conforms to the second, recommended principle: it is low in fat, and excludes the consumption of salt-cured, salt-pickled, and smoked foods. It is also low fat and encourages "the frequent consumption of certain fruits and vegetables." No diet can be termed a sure cancer-prevention diet at this time; but within these limited principles, D.D. can be called an *anti-cancer diet*.

The National Research Council Report also makes a vital point about the need to reduce food intake:

> . . . the committee concluded that neither the epidemiological studies [human] nor the experiments in animals permit a clear interpretation of the specific effect of total caloric intake on the risk of cancer. Nevertheless, the studies conducted in animals show that a reduction in total food intake decreases the age-specific incidence of cancer. The evidence is less clear for human beings.

In respect to consumption of *fats*, the report states:

> Epidemiological [human] studies have repeatedly shown an association between dietary fat and the occurrence of cancer at various sites, especially the breast, prostate, and large bowel. In various populations, both the high incidence of and mortality from breast cancer have been shown to correlate strongly with higher per capita fat consumption; the few case-control studies conducted have also shown this association with dietary fat.
>
> Like breast cancer, increased risk of large-bowel cancer has been associated with higher fat intake in both correlation and case-control studies. The data on prostate cancer are limited, but they too suggest that an increased risk is related to high levels of dietary fat. In general, it is not possible to identify specific components of fat as being clearly respon-

sible for the observed effects, although total fatand saturated fat have been associated most frequently.

Concerning numerous experiments with animals regarding the effects of *fats* on cancer, the report reveals:
An increase in fat intake from 5% to 20% of the weight of the diet (i.e., approximately 10% to 40% of total calories) increases tumor incidence in various tissues; conversely, animals consuming low-fat diets have a lower tumor incidence.

The report stresses that:
It is not now possible, and may never be possible on the basis of current evidence, to formulate interim dietary guidelines that are consistent with good nutritional practices and likely to reduce the risk of cancer.

We condensed these conclusions to the following primary guidelines for your food and beverage consumption:

- Cut down fat intake.
- Include fruits, vegetables, and whole-wheat grain cereal products in the daily diet.
- Minimize consumption of food preserved by salt-curing, salt-pickling, and smoking.
- Excessive consumption of alcoholic beverages should be avoided, particularly when combined with cigarette smoking. If alcoholic beverages are consumed, they should be used in moderation.

The directions for the Delicious Quick-Trim Diet embody all these vital points. We must emphasize that the National Research Council has not read nor has any connection with this book. Please note that the excellent complete report, "Diet, Nutrition, and Cancer," is available at reasonable cost from National Academy Press, 2101 Constitution Ave., N.W., Washington DC 20418.

Many other studies relate fat and overweight with cancer. Dr. N. F. Boyd of the Ontario Cancer Institute in Toronto has reported that "the risk of developing breast cancer is known to increase with increasing overweight," and that the overall mortality rate of overweight patients was "significantly reduced" when they reduced their overweight.

In a continuing study of more than a million people from 1959 to the present, Dr. Boyd has reported that, "Being too fat increases risk of cancer of the breast and gall bladder,` and of uterine and ovarian cancer in women; of colon-rectal and prostate cancer in men." In an article in *The New York Times*, Dr. Arthur Upton of the National Cancer Institute recommended that Americans should eat less fat, drink less alcohol, eat more dietary fiber from fresh fruits, vegetables, and cereals—and avoid being overweight to reduce the possible risk of cancer. Alcohol, he said, is associated with a high risk of digestive-tract and liver cancers, and should be held to one or two drinks a day.

The May 29, 1982, issue of *The Lancet*, an internationally respected British medical journal, spotlighted:

the positive correlation between body weight and cancer. . . . The link was established from actuarial records over forty years ago and has held up consistently ever since. Figures published in 1960 from the Metropolitan Life Insurance Company of New York, for example, showed that men had a 16% and women a 13% excess mortality from cancer if they were 20% or more above their ideal weight.

Founder and president of the American Health Foundation, Dr. Ernst L. Wynder has stated, "We now have evidence that an overall lowering in fat is helpful to reduction in atherosclerosis and cancers of the breast, prostate, colon cancer and possibly pancreas."

In the authoritative work *Toward the Conquest of Cancer*, Dr. Edward J. Beattie, Jr., Chief Medical Officer and General Director of Memorial Hospital, at the Memorial Sloan-Kettering Cancer Center, has written (with coauthor Stuart D. Cowan), "What we eat, and do not eat, plays an important, indirect role in causing and preventing cancer."

Michael F. Jacobson, Executive Director of the Center for Science in the Public Interest, has said, "Of all the problems that have been identified in foods in recent years . . . fat is far and away the number one problem."

In case there is any confusion, we must clarify that none of the quotations and references in this cancer section were made specifically about the Delicious Quick-Trim Diets. The fact is that the D.D. guidelines were created deliberately to coincide with all the principles stated by these and many other authorities.

THE QUESTION OF CHOLESTEROL

CHOLESTEROL has become a scare word for many people, but it is a normal component of blood and tissues, found in every animal cell. Some cholesterol is synthesized by the body, and some is supplied by what we eat. The amounts vary according to the types and amounts of foods we ingest.

TRIGLYCERIDES derive from "a compound (ester) linking three molecules of fatty acids," and are another normal element of blood and tissues.

There is some confusion and disagreement in the scientific world about both, but there is general agreement that too much or too little cholesterol can be harmful. There is little question that the amount of cholesterol in the foods one eats is related positively to the amount of cholesterol in the blood.

The health benefits, notably the *life-saving* results, of low-cholesterol and low-triglyceride eating, have been demonstrated in a controlled study in Norway. Over 1,200 men, aged forty to forty-nine, who had high levels of blood cholesterol, were involved. Some switched to special low-cholesterol, low-triglyceride eating—while others continued eating as before.

After five years, the dieting group averaged 13 percent lower blood cholesterol than the others, had considerably lower triglyceride levels—and experienced a sharp reduction in heart attacks and heart-related deaths. Smoking also made an important difference, but the diet benefits alone were dramatically significant.

The only sure and intelligent way for you to maintain a healthful balance of both factors is to have your doctor conduct laboratory tests that reveal your personal cholesterol and triglyceride counts. He will advise you on treatment and diet.

The National Research Council states that: "The relationship between dietary cholesterol and cancer is not clear. . . . Data on cholesterol and cancer risk from studies in animals are too limited to permit any inferences to be drawn." There is general agreement, however, that a high cholesterol level increases the chances of coronary heart disease and stroke. Other influencing elements are the foods you eat, overweight, high blood pressure, diabetes, family history, physical inertia, and cigarette smoking. All, including cholesterol and triglycerides, may be related to the development of *arteriosclerosis*, an arterial disease characterized by a hardening and thickening of the artery walls, with lessened blood flow. It's not difficult to imagine how the kind of eating that makes for overweight—rich in calories and high in cholesterol and saturated fats—would contribute to a hardening of the arteries or to heart disease.

*Once again, Delicious Quick-Trim Diets are not only low in calories, but also low in cholesterol and triglycerides.*They are also low in saturated and unsaturated fat, both of which may have an important effect on your health. *Saturated fats*, usually derived from animal tissue, become solid at room temperatures or lower (like the congealed fat you've seen on plates with fatty meats); these tend to raise cholesterol levels.

Unsaturated fats, vegetable fats, including polyunsaturated oils and margarine, are usually liquid at room temperature, aid in reducing blood cholesterol, and contain no cholesterol. But . . . *this is vital in reducing: The vegetable, unsaturated fats are very high in calories—just one tablespoon of polyunsaturated vegetable oil is 125 calories.*

Here are the two basic rules to follow in this area:

1. To help control *cholesterol*, limit your consumption of *high-fat* foods.
2. To help control *triglycerides*, limit your consumption of *high-carbohydrate* foods.

Fats and oils are mostly triglycerides, not cholesterol. This is apparent in the table that follows, where the foods highest in cholesterol (that is, egg yolk, liver, and kidney) are not most fatty (that is, cream, butter, and cream cheese).

Be wary of *hidden saturated fats*—read ingredients carefully on packages and check for content of saturated fats and oils. Those to beware of include coconut oil (rather than vegetable oils), lard, animal fats, palm and olive oils.

The following partial list shows you the great differences in cholesterol content among common foods and beverages (for a complete listing, check the *Composition of Foods* Agriculture Handbook no. 8, and no. 456, USDA, available in libraries).

FOOD AND AMOUNT	CHOLESTEROL (milligrams)
Milk, skim or buttermilk, 1 cup	5
Milk, whole, 1 cup (note that whole milk has almost seven times the cholesterol content of skim milk or buttermilk)	34

FOOD AND AMOUNT	CHOLESTEROL (milligrams)
Cream, light table, 1 fl. oz.	20
Cottage cheese, uncreamed, ½ cup	7
Cottage cheese, creamed, ½ cup	24
Yogurt, low-fat, plain, ½ cup	9
Butter, 1 tbs.	35
Egg, whole or yolk alone	250
Egg, white only	0
Ice cream, ½ cup	27
Ice milk, ½ cup	13
Cheese, Cheddar, 1 oz.	28
Cheese, cream, 1 oz.	31
Mayonnaise, 1 tbs.	8
Chicken, turkey, lt. meat, 3 oz., cooked	67
Chicken, turkey, dark meat, 3 oz., cooked	77
Beef, lean, 3 oz., cooked	75
Liver, beef or calf, 3 oz., cooked	370
Kidney, 3 oz., cooked	680
Lamb, lean, 3 oz., cooked	85
Veal, lean, 3 oz., cooked	84
Pork, lean, 3 oz., cooked	75
Ham, boiled, lean, 3 oz.	75
Salmon, canned, 3 oz.	30
Salmon, cooked, 3 oz.	40
Halibut cooked, 3 oz.	40
Flounder, cooked, 3 oz.	69
Mackerel, cooked, 3 oz.	84
Tuna, canned, reg., 3 oz.	55
Lobster, 3 oz., cooked	75
Shrimp, 3 oz., cooked	130

DATA ON DIETARY FIBER

Dietary fiber is a combination of complex carbohydrates, such as cellulose and other compounds that make up the cell walls and structural formations in plants. Examples are stems of salad greens, celery, apple skins, wheat bran, and various other fruits.

"Crude fiber" represents as little as one seventh of the total dietary fiber in food, and need not concern us here.

The primary value of dietary fiber in the food you eat is in helping to relieve and control constipation. That's a considerable benefit, making it worthwhile to eat—*but not overeat*—high-fiber, high-bulk foods. Many fiber-containing foods—fruits, vegetables, and cereals—are included in Delicious Quick-Trim Diets in sufficient quantity for the adult in normal health. Drinking plenty of water, particularly with meals, improves the effect of dietary fiber, which swells as it absorbs water, adding bulk. This greater bulk promotes regularity in elimination. It also contributes to a feeling of fullness when reducing.

Fruits, particularly with the skins, contain sizable amounts of dietary fiber, as do raw and cooked vegetables. Fruits with seeds, such as strawberries, raspberries, blackberries, and kiwis are fine sources of fiber, too. Cereals and breads made from whole wheat have more fiber content than those made with refined wheat, which has had the bran (the partly ground husk) removed.

Despite claims by some zealots that "fiber" in foods is a health miracle, it is only one component, neither magical nor all curative. The fact is that fiber foods such as breads and cereals are relatively high in calories, and should be consumed within limitations, as specified by D.D. Guidelines. The Delicious Diets provide plenty of other fiber foods, such as vegetables, that are lower in calories. This is in line with a policy statement of the Institute of Food Technologists' Expert Panel on Food Safety and Nutrition, which maintains that

> Recommendations regarding the consumption of any nu-
> trient must be rational and based on reasonable scientific
> evidence. In the absence of such evidence, *moderation* should
> be exercised. A variety of whole-grain products, fruits, and
> vegetables will ensure a good mixture of fiber constituents,
> and make a positive contribution to the overall nutritional
> value of the diet.

There is agreement that your daily meals should include some dietary fiber, but there's no question that too much fiber can be harmful. For one thing, ingesting too much fiber can interfere with proper absorption of vital minerals, such as calcium, iron, and zinc, and can lead to a health problem. "Everything in excess," it has been stated wisely, "is opposed to nature."

Among the dietary fiber foods you may eat on D.D. (within the daily guidelines) are the following, which are relatively high in fiber:

Vegetables

Broccoli, boiled, drained, ½ inch pcs., ½ cup	3.2
Brussels sprouts, boiled, drained, ½ cup	2.3
Cabbage, shredded, boiled, drained, ½ cup	2.0
Carrots, sliced, boiled, drained, ½ cup	2.3
Eggplant, peeled, diced, cooked, drained, ½ cup	2.5
Green beans, cut, boiled, ½ cup	2.0
Lettuce, ⅙ head	1.4
Okra, ½ cup	2.6
Spinach, boiled, drained, ½ cup	5.7
Tomato, raw, medium	2.0
Turnips, boiled, mashed, ½ cup	3.2

Fruits

Apple, with peel, medium	3.3
Banana, medium	4.0
Honeydew melon, medium wedge	1.3
Nectarine, medium	3.0
Orange, medium	3.0
Pear, medium	3.0
Raspberries, ½ cup	4.6
Strawberries, ½ cup	1.7

Cereals

All Bran, ⅓ cup (1 oz.)	9.0
Bran flakes, 40%, ⅔ cup (1 oz.)	4.0

Breads

Cracked-wheat, 1 slice	2.1
Whole-wheat, 1 slice	2.1

Whatever you are eating, high-fiber foods or otherwise, if at any time you have any disturbing change in your bowel habits (constipation, diarrhea, etc.), the condition should be checked with your physician.

MAKING SENSE ABOUT SALT/SODIUM

Throughout this book there have been many references to restricting the use of salt (sodium chloride). Overuse is particularly undesirable when reducing, since sodium holds water within the system, adding weight. Salt can be dangerous to your health in other ways, too.

Of primary importance to you right now is the fact that *Delicious Quick-Trim Diets are low in salt intake.* If your doctor has advised you to restrict your salt intake severely because of personal health problems, be guided by his instructions.

Some salt is essential in the human diet, but just how much is needed? It has been estimated that the minimum daily requirement for sodium is about 200 milligrams (half a gram of salt)—though some authorities suggest that as little as 25 to 50 milligrams of sodium a day is preferable (.06 to .12 grams of salt).

How much do most individuals ingest? In shocking contrast, it is estimated that the average American daily intake of salt is 10 to 12 grams. That's 5 to 6 teaspoons, or—almost 20 pounds of salt a year per person.

While it's difficult, perhaps impossible, to figure your own salt intake, it's probable that you, like most people today, ingest too much—and that may become harmful to you. While each individual's requirements vary, those with high blood pressure (hypertension) are especially vulnerable to salt's injurious effects.

It's estimated that one out of five persons in the world is afflicted with hypertension, some 25 million or more individuals in the United States alone. That is a matter of serious concern for all of us. While it has not been scientifically proven that salt intake *causes* hypertension, that premise is pretty much accepted.

If one has hypertension, blood pressure usually drops when salt use is severely restricted. It rises again when a good deal of salt is consumed. In addition, there is a definite relationship between obesity (as well as hypertension) and high salt intake.

As stated before, a minimal amount of salt is essential to human functioning, and we usually get plenty of sodium compounds that exist naturally in everyday foods. That includes fish, meat, poultry, vegetables, dairy products—even drinking water from the tap, wells, brooks, and rivers. Naturally or artificially carbonated waters also tend to contain sodium.

Here's a list showing approximate amounts of salt contained in some everyday foods. The second list indicates the approximate amounts of salt in some commercial and processed products:

FOOD AND AMOUNT	SALT/SODIUM (milligrams)
Beets, cut up, 1 cup	70
Broccoli, cooked, cut up, 1 cup	14
Cabbage, cooked, 1 cup	20

285

FOOD AND AMOUNT	SALT/SODIUM (milligrams)
Carrots, cut up, 1 cup	50
Celery, cut up, 1 cup	130
Cantaloupe, half	10
Cauliflower, cooked, 1 cup	12
Egg, 1 large	60
Milk, whole, 1 cup (skim milk, similar)	135
Radishes, 1 cup	16
Spinach, cooked, 1 cup	80
Turnips, cut up, 1 cup	50
Watercress, 1 cup	50
Processed and Commercial	
Bread, white, 1 slice	150
Catsup, 1 tbs.	150
Cookies, average size	100–300
Cornflakes, ½ cup	125
Cupcake, medium size	200–300
Fish, fast food, fried, average portion	800
Frankfurter, 1, 5" long	600
Green beans, canned, 1 cup	550
Hamburger, fast food, average size	700
Italian dressing, bottled, 1 tbs.	300
Mustard, prepared, 1 tbs.	200
Olives, pickled, green, 6 large	570
Olives, ripe, 6 large	200
Peanut butter, 1 tbs.	100
Pickle, dill, 1 medium	900
Pie, apple, average slice	400
Pizza, 2-oz. portion	300–500
Sauerkraut, 1 cup	1,700
Soup, bean and pork, canned, 1 cup	2,100
Soy sauce, 1 tbs.	1,300
Tomatoes, canned, 1 cup	300

While these lists are not all-inclusive and figures are by necessity approximate, we can learn a great deal by making comparisons. Note, for example, the sizable difference between fresh and canned vegetables.

When you eat or drink products labeled "no sodium added," "low sodium," or "no salt added," the food may still contain some sodium naturally—but the reduction in your salt intake will be considerable and highly desirable. There is sodium, too, in many medications, such as prescription drugs, over-the-counter antacids (sodium bicarbonate, etc.), and analgesics like aspirin.

Don't overlook the Delicious possibilities (detailed in earlier chapters) of using seasonings that are flavorful but nonsodium. Instead of salt, consider using herbs, spices, no-salt seasonings, chives, garlic, lime, lemons, and other tasty ingredients. Since they're used in small quantities, any sodium content becomes negligible. Avoid *overuse* of "salt substitutes," which may contain potentially harmful ingredients if ingested in large amounts over a period of time.

As a person in normal health, be wary but not overanxious or fanatical about avoiding salt. Don't be turned away from other desirable and essential value in many foods, such as unprocessed vegetables, poultry, fish, and many other edibles in spite of some sodium content. You couldn't survive without any sodium whatsoever.

The central point here is that for your greatest health and long-life potential, medical science advises you to keep your salt intake to a sensible minimum. Don't oversalt foods in cooking or at the table. Avoid salt-cured, salt-pickled, smoked, and highly salted foods.

In short, do be cautious but don't be irrational in your use of salt. Tests have shown, as we noted earlier, that individuals denied added salt since infancy never missed its taste or flavor. Salting of food is an acquired taste. Once you cut down, you'll probably develop a distaste for oversalted foods. And you'll find it a lot easier to slim down and stay trim.

SUGAR—HOW SWEET IT ISN'T

Doctors may still question the relationship between sugar overconsumption and various health problems, but medical science is *certain* that sugar is high in calories and that overconsumption of sugar *contributes specifically to overweight and obesity.*

As we have noted, obesity is spotlighted as increasing the risk of heart disease, hypertension, diabetes—and has been linked with possible contributing involvement in a number of other ailments, such as dental decay. While carbohydrates, including sugars, are essential to the diet in some degree, keep in mind that every teaspoon of sugar alone adds about 16 calories to everything else you eat.

Ingesting a lot of high-sugar foods tends to displace other, more nutritious foods, so sugar not only contributes to excess weight, but also interferes with a healthy, balanced diet.

Sugars are "simple" carbohydrates that provide calories but few nutrients, and are therefore often referred to as "empty calories." In contrast, vegetables and fruits, along with basic cereals and other starches, are "complex" carbohydrates. They supply some vitamins, minerals, and other nutritious elements along with bulk.

Lest you be concerned that you may be depriving yourself of needed sugar, please understand that you get some sugar *naturally* from fruits, vegetables, and other foods within D.D. Guidelines.

In addition to cookies, cakes, candies, ice cream, sodas, and other obviously sugary items, sugar is contained in most cereals, bread, canned and bottled foods, cured meats, frozen foods, and on and on. The sugar content in ready-to-eat cereals ranges from over 50 percent of the total dry weight to less than 1 percent. So, as with many other foods, you have a choice. It's important to your health and weight control to be selective.

The usual 12-ounce can of soda contains about 7 to 9 teaspoons of sugar. That adds 112 to 144 calories to your daily calories-IN-calories-OUT stay-trim control equation—all of them on the calories-IN side of the scale. Beware of sugary soda if you want to be slim; here again you do have Delicious sugar-free alternatives.

All sugars have about the same number of calories: common granulated sugar, cane sugar, beet sugar, honey, molasses, maple sugar, glucose, dextrose, sucrose, turbinado sugar, brown sugar, milk sugar, and maltose. Don't be misled by high-priced "health sugars"—the only real difference between them and ordinary sugar is the cost. Ask any objective physician or chemist.

You cut down on your sugar intake automatically and healthfully when you observe D.D. Guidelines. Aside from that, we urge you to stop spooning sugar into coffee, tea, cereals, and other foods. Seek no-sugar-added fruits such as pineapple (fresh or packed in its own juice), and other sugar-free foods and beverages. All are readily available. Moderate use of artificial sweeteners and artificially sweetened items is generally permissible.

Finally, there is no need to become frantic about sugar use—unless you have some medical problem and your doctor has advised you to keep sugar intake to an absolute minimum. Do cut down however, while you lose pounds and inches following D.D. directions.

SENSIBLE VIEWS ON VITAMINS AND MINERALS

As an adult in normal health (if you're not, you shouldn't be on any diet without your doctor's approval), you'll get enough vitamins and minerals on your Delicious Diet. If you wish to take a once-daily, all-purpose vitamin-mineral tablet, go ahead—it may be helpful.

We recommend to you this statement by the U.S. Food and Drug Administration (FDA): "Your body not only needs vitamins and other nutrients, it needs the bulk and textures of real foods."

The following vitamins are contained (though not necessarily in total daily requirements) in the real foods you are eating on your Delicious Quick-Trim Diet: Vitamins A (retinol), B^1 (thiamine), B^6 (pyridoxine, pyridoxal, pyridoxamine), B^2 (riboflavin), B^{12} (cyanocobalamin), C (ascorbic acid), D (calciferol), E (tocopherols), K, biotin, folic acid (folacin), niacin, pantothenic acid, plus traces of others.

Our purpose here is to help you reduce most effectively, not to get into minute details and controversy about vitamins and minerals. But there are a few basic facts about vitamins and minerals you should know:

1. *Are additional vitamin and mineral products needed?* Only your doctor can determine your individual needs. The FDA states:

> While vitamins are essential for good health, excessive amounts are unnecessary and may be harmful. . . . Foods can and do supply most Americans with adequate nutrients, and consumers should not expect any major physical benefits from multivitamin pills, contrary to the myth.

The FDA notes further:

> As research continues, there will be more answers as to how much is too much of a vitamin, what the entire scope of usefulness of each vitamin is, and which medical conditions may respond well to vitamin therapy. In the meantime, consumers should know that elaborate testimonials, miraculous claims, and vitamins supposedly derived from exotic sources

result from mere guesswork, confusion, and often, outright fraud.

2. *What about "natural" versus synthetic (processed) vitamins and minerals?*

Again, here's the viewpoint of the U.S. Food and Drug Administration:

> Each vitamin has a particular molecular structure that remains the same whether it's synthesized in a laboratory or extracted from an animal or plant or consumed as part of an animal or plant. To be called "vitamin A," for example, there has to be a specific molecular arrangement that is identical no matter where it is found or how it is derived. The body cannot distinguish in any way from a vitamin from a plant or animal and the same vitamin from a laboratory.

Consider the warning from a notable biochemist at the University of Texas Medical Branch: "I wouldn't be surprised to see some new diseases arising—not from vitamin deficiencies this time, but rather from vitamin excesses."

If you wish to take extra vitamins and minerals while on D.D. or Nutri-Maintenance Eating, we recommend moderation again. Whatever benefits you may get from vitamins and minerals, realize that they don't replace nutritious, low-fat eating. As Dr. William Castelli, director of the long-established Framingham, Massachusetts, heart study program, points out, "If people think they can go out and eat all the hamburgers and hot dogs they want and be safe by taking vitamin B^6, they're crazy."

DATA ON DIETARY MINERALS

There's no question that dietary minerals—those that the body can use beneficially—are also essential in the diet. Some minerals are needed in relatively large amounts—"large" being measured in terms of milligrams. Each milligram is only one thousandth of a gram, and a gram equals 0.035 ounce. The main dietary minerals are calcium, chloride, magnesium, phosphorus, potassium, and sulfur.

"Trace minerals" are needed only in extremely small quantities. They include cobalt, copper, fluorine, iodine, iron, manganese, selenium, zinc, perhaps others.

290

Not all minerals are beneficial to the human system. Some—including cadmium, mercury, and lead—may be extremely harmful.

The dosage of minerals you ingest should be controlled specifically by a knowledgeable physician, according to your individual needs. A potassium deficiency, for example, may render you severely weak and ill; on the other hand, an overdose of potassium can trigger serious disorders. The same is true of other minerals as well as some vitamins. Ingesting as little as twice as much as you need for good health may bring on adverse effects.

CALCIUM is present in the body in greater amounts than any other mineral. It's especially vital to the bones and teeth. Growing children and pregnant and lactating women have the greatest need for calcium. There are strong indications that calcium deficiency may contribute to high blood pressure. Calcium is present in many foods—milk and milk products (cottage cheese, for example), green leafy vegetables, and citrus fruits. Among foods especially high in calcium are canned sardines (drained of oil) and salmon with bones, skim milk, yogurt, oysters, and creamed cottage cheese.

POTASSIUM, which helps regulate body fluids and volume, is abundant in almost all foods, both plant and animal. If you take a diuretic, your doctor has probably recommended extra potassium, particularly from bananas and orange juice, plus prescribed medication if necessary. Other foods containing potassium are apples, apricots, asparagus, blackberries, cantaloupe, chicken, honeydew melon, milk, mushrooms, oranges, plums, beet greens, broccoli, grapefruit, raw carrots, spinach, canned tuna, and tomatoes.

An adequate diet of varied foods normally supplies sufficient potassium.

CHLORIDE AND SODIUM, which combine to form table salt (sodium chloride) are essential for good health, but overconsumption in daily eating can have ill effects, as previously noted. You get plenty of sodium naturally in animal products primarily—poultry, fish, meat, milk and milk products, eggs. There's lots of sodium, often too much, in processed foods. For good health and long life, one basic rule is to avoid oversalting your system.

PHOSPHORUS is needed for bones and teeth, in about the same

proportions as calcium. You will normally get enough phosphorus through a regular, varied diet, particularly from poultry, whole-grain foods, and eggs.

MAGNESIUM is found principally in the bones, and in all body tissues. A deficiency is seldom present in individuals eating a normal varied diet, only in certain disease and alcoholic situations. Magnesium is ingested in the usual diet through consumption of fish, raw greens in salads, whole-grain foods, milk and milk products, meats, and nuts such as almonds and cashews.

SULFUR, present in all body tissues, is essential to human life, but its complete function has not been established. As a component of several important amino acids, it is part of two vitamins, biotin and thiamine. It is rarely related to deficiencies in human beings in a civilized society, since sulfur is contained in many protein foods, including fish, poultry, and meat.

TRACE MINERALS OR ELEMENTS are essential to human functioning, but are present in the body in extremely small amounts. Possible deficiencies in iron, zinc, and others should be checked carefully by laboratory tests. Most of these minerals are present in varied foods eaten normally, such as poultry, fish, meat, green leafy vegetables, whole-grain products, eggs and nuts.

Remember, both the Delicious Basic Diet and Delicious Variety Diet supply enough of the desirable vitamins, minerals, and trace elements for the normally healthy person. Just follow the menus and directions given throughout this book.

THE CAFFEINE CONFLICT

It's important to admit that at this writing, the long debate about whether caffeine—consumed primarily in coffee, tea, and soft drinks—is injurious to humans has yet to be resolved. Animal studies have revealed some harmful effects, but any direct relationship between these results and human consumption has not yet been proved.

Dr. Sanford Miller, Director of the FDA Bureau of Foods, has described coffee as "a potent, biologically active material." One of the prime directives of physicians to individuals who have heart problems, ulcers, and certain other ailments is to stop intake of regular coffee, tea, and any beverages or products containing caffeine. The same is usually true in respect to pregnant women. If coffee causes indigestion or stomach upset, avoid it.

Here is the most up-to-date medical opinion on the use of caffeine by normally healthy individuals:

- Don't drink more than one or two cups of regular coffee daily.
- Limit the drinking of regular tea to one to three cups a day.
- It's preferable to avoid caffeine-containing cola drinks, particularly for growing children.
- Limit the use of nonprescription drugs that contain a sizable amount of caffeine—usually diet pills, some combination analgesics, and certain cold pills (always check labels for caffeine content).

How much coffee is needed to overstimulate or lead to sleeplessness is very much an individual effect. You alone can decide for yourself, depending on your personal reaction. When cutting down or giving up coffee, some people experience severe withdrawal symptoms, while others report minimal effects.

The most recent laboratory results reveal these caffeine levels, measured in milligrams:

Coffee (5 ounces): Regular—automatic drip, 110 to 150; percolated, 64 to 124; instant, 40 to 108; decaffeinated brewed, 2 to 5; decaffeinated instant, 2.

Tea (5 ounces): Brewed 5 minutes, 20 to 50; 3 mins., 20 to 46; 1 min., 9 to 33; 12 ounces iced-tea can, 22 to 36. According to a study on the effect of brewing time on caffeine content in tea, over 50 percent of the caffeine (after a 5-minute brewing time) was released in the first minute. Decaffeinated tea and herbal teas contain minimal amounts of caffeine.

Soda (12 ounces): Cola, regular or diet cola, 33 to 52. Colas and other soft drinks without caffeine are now available; look for "no caffeine" or "caffeine-free" on cans and bottles.

Nonprescription drugs, usual dose: "diet pills," 200 to 280; combination pain relievers, 64 to 130; diuretics, 100 to 200; stimulants (combating sleepiness), 200.

To cut down on caffeine in coffee, some people enjoy a mixture of regular and decaffeinated coffees—either instant or brewed.

(Brewed decaffeinated coffee is generally more tasteful than instant.) Many people serve brewed decaffeinated coffee without mentioning it; most say that guests compliment the coffee without realizing that they are drinking decaffeinated. Others add a spoonful of ground espresso coffee to decaffeinated grind for stronger flavor.

A dash of anisette or other liqueur enlivens the flavor of decaffeinated coffee. (More than a dash dominates the flavor and adds too many calories.) Decaffeinated espresso (double-roast), either ground or instant, is available at some stores. An increasing number of fine restaurants offer brewed decaffeinated coffee, much preferred by most patrons over instant coffee packets.

ARE "HEALTH FOODS" MORE HEALTHFUL?

Are so-called "health foods" and "organic" produce—foods usually sold in health food stores or by mail order, truly aids to better health and longer life? Are the claims supported by scientific evidence? Accredited scientists and most physicians we have questioned believe they are not. Certainly such offerings are usually higher in price than comparable food store items—often to a shockingly inflated degree. Furthermore, claims that fruits and vegetables are "organic" (grown without chemical fertilizers or pesticides) are often unverifiable. Many "organic gardeners" and "naturalists" use compost composed of animal manure, entrails, and rotted garbage to grow their produce, yet they condemn scientifically formulated chemical fertilizers that have been proven safe, healthful, and effective in innumerable tests by agricultural and university laboratories.

A report by a panel of forty-eight scientists with no known financial ties to food and chemical industries stated:

Natural products may now be label-free, but they definitely are not free of chemicals, sugar, fats, and cholesterol. If labeled, potatoes would be shown to contain 150 different chemical substances, including 24 hydrocarbons, 24 kinds of alcohol, 31 carbonyls, 13 acids, 9 bases, and 23 sulphur compounds.

They state that because such natural products are label-free the myth is perpetuated that there are "poisons" in processed foods, but not in natural ones. Shoppers should be aware, however, that all potatoes contain arsenic, that all lima beans have traces of hydrogen cyanide, and that all carrots contain the hallucinogen myristicin.

The significant point here is that potatoes, lima beans, and carrots are all nutritious foods, of course, *despite* chemical ingredients that tend to frighten the unknowing.

Be well informed, and you can avoid being taken in by questionable or false claims in the guise of "nutrition." Be on guard against those self-serving zealots who try to scare people with the alarmingly negative point of view that "living itself is dangerous to your health"—some of them in order to profit personally by selling their own products.

Be wary of narrowly focused, self-designated "experts" who disparage others with terms like "junk food" and "fad diet" in order to advance their own interests. It's much easier to use derogatory phrases than to supply clear, scientifically objective information. I've encountered a number of "experts" who automatically condemn any diet or diet book they themselves haven't created—*especially if they haven't read the book.*

CAUTIONS ON EATING WHEN TRAVELING

When you travel to most large cities and resorts, you can eat as you would at home, safely and healthfully, within D.D. and Nutri-Maintenance Guidelines. The cautions here are to be observed mostly when traveling in more primitive areas, where sanitary conditions may be questionable. The points are worth keeping in mind wherever you travel—use your good sense and be wary rather than excessively worried.

- Avoid an excess of rich gravies, creamy sauces, and fatty dressings. When refrigeration is doubtful, fats—including butter, oils, and lard—may have been exposed for lengthy periods in warmth. Thus harmful bacteria may be present, multiplying rapidly. Lack of sanitary personal care by individuals preparing and serving food could increase the danger of contamination.

- Don't indulge heavily in exotic foods to which your stomach is not accustomed—overspiced, oversauced dishes. While eating just a little of such food may be tolerated, your system may rebel against sizable quantities, resulting in severe indigestion, nausea, or worse.
- If your stomach is upset, limit consumption of alcoholic drinks, which may tend to aggravate rather than soothe the condition.
- Be guarded against rich, creamy dishes like custards, puddings, and pies. If left in a warm place, a culture medium is created, inviting the growth of staphylococcus and other germs.
- In many areas of the world, it's wise to drink only bottled water that has not come from the tap. Carbonated sodas may be safer. If the water is suspect, it's wise to avoid salads and fruits that have been washed in that water. When ordering hot or iced tea or coffee, try to make sure that the water has been *boiled*, not just heated. Keep in mind also that ice and ice cubes in drinks may be contaminated.
- Well-cooked meats, poultry, and fish are safer than those which are rare, particularly in places where refrigeration, storage, and sanitation may be inadequate.
- Foods that are well broiled, baked, or boiled are generally safer than exotic and creamy dishes.
- Be cautious about buying any edibles from sidewalk vendors. Peel raw fruit and vegetables beforehand if you're going to eat them uncooked. Unpeeled bananas are safe.
- It takes little room to pack one-serving packets of oatmeal, instant broth, decaffeinated coffee, and any other nonfatty foods you can eat or drink by adding boiling water when available. If you're feeling too ill to eat solid foods, these packets can be a great aid to your quick recovery. Plain bread is a safe food; learn to order "bread without butter" in local languages.
- To maintain your good health and enjoy every possible minute of your trip, *never overload your system by eating or drinking too much*. It's a fact in travel groups that if most of the people have severe indigestion, dysentery, and other upsets, those who stay well are likely to have eaten lightly while the others have filled up or overstuffed.

It's always true that a small portion of a fine-tasting food has the same delectable flavor as a heaping plateful. And it's a lot safer if the food's contaminated.

- NOTE: We realize that half the joy of travel is experiencing new and different things, including native food and drinks. And we don't mean to restrict your fun. We owe it to your health to list these cautions—the rest is up to you. Happy traveling!
- *When you return* from your travels, if you step on the scale (as you should) and discover you have gained weight, please don't waste time and emotional energy feeling guilty about it. Go right back on your Delicious Diet—or perhaps on the One-Day Liquid Diet, or the Three-Day Vegetable Diet, as you choose. By the next morning the scale will score you as a pound or more lighter. In a matter of days you'll be back down to your desired weight and slim figure once more.

ANOREXIA NERVOSA? BULIMIA?

This brief review may clear up some of the confusion and mis-understanding about the "wasting disease," *anorexia nervosa* ("nervous loss of appetite" . . . "an hysterical condition"), an extremely complicated and largely unresolved illness. Our main purpose in this discussion is to emphasize the urgent need for medical treatment. Immediate professional care is essential, since an obsession toward starvation and extreme thinness can carry one to the edge of death, and sometimes does prove fatal.

Points generally agreed upon by authorities are: Most anorexics are younger than twenty-five years of age. Over 90 percent are women, overwhelmingly in the upper- and middle-income categories. Nothing could be more fallacious than the popular notion that anorexia nervosa is a disease of overweights trying to reduce. A comprehensive study noted that "Most anorexics are no more than ten pounds overweight when they begin to diet, and some are not overweight at all." A further consensus is that *anorexia nervosa* is not just an eating disorder but a disorder of the whole person.

Although anorexia nervosa has been in the spotlight in recent years, the disease is not new; in fact, it has been around for centuries. Cases were recorded as far back as in the 1600s.

The current focus on anorexia nervosa is valuable in order to keep people alert to possible danger when an individual becomes excessively thin and still keeps rejecting food. The anorexic starves by choice and compulsion, with no will to be treated or cured. If you suspect that anyone in the family or otherwise is an anorexic, seek experienced medical attention and explore the possibility of psychiatric therapy.

Bulimia (bulemia, boulimea) is a similar sickness, differing in specific respects. Most of these afflicted persons go on eating sprees or binges, ingesting masses of food, then forcing themselves to throw up in order not to gain weight. This illness can also be serious, even deadly, and requires speedy medical treatment and therapy. It too is an emotional affliction, *a disorder of the whole person.*

MUST EX-SMOKERS GAIN WEIGHT?

If you are a cigarette smoker, you know the indicated health dangers—cancer of the lungs and other areas, heart disease, emphysema, and other serious ills. Our purpose here is not to scare you into giving up cigarettes, but to try to help you to reduce if you're overweight, and to help keep you from piling on excess pounds—whether you're a smoker or not.

It's a fact that many people put on weight after they snuff out what they determine is their last cigarette. Certainly some iron-willed individuals quit, never smoke again, and don't put on an extra pound. But not everyone can do that.

If you're overweight and determined to reduce *and* stop smoking cigarettes, realize that few can or should do both at the same time. Changing both eating and smoking habits simultaneously becomes a double strain that can sometimes bring on emotional problems. It's your decision, but we must sound this note of caution—for your total health.

If you tackle your smoking problem first, you may be able to manage more effectively, taking it as the first step of your twin-powered program—to achieve optimum health and longer life.

If you decide to slim down to your desired weight first, you now know that you can reduce within a relatively short time—the length of time depending on how overweight you are. On D.D., you have the decisive advantage that you cut down on calories *and* enjoy Delicious flavor too, as never possible before.

Then you continue to take pleasure in exceptionally delectable eating as you stay beautifully trim on Nutri-Maintenance Eating. Once slim as desired, you may then be able to stop smoking with greater determination and confidence.

Why do many smokers, women and men, gain weight when they give up cigarettes? There is general agreement among many authorities on the typical profile—a woman in this example. By temperament or conditioning, she tends to satisfy her *oral* desires. Consciously or not, she gets some of this gratification from smoking cigarettes.

When she stops smoking, she seeks a substitute—generally not realizing it. Usually she tries to satisfy her oral cravings with candy, chewing gum, sweets, extra eating, and snacking, often repeatedly day and night. The pounds and inches pile on, making her increasingly unhappy and irritable due to giving up her smoking habit, perhaps ingrained over many years.

For many people, cigarette smoking can act to curb the appetite, also serving at times as a food substitute. Instead of taking a coffee break with a cup of coffee and a cigarette, she stuffs her mouth with a pastry. The same can be true at lunch, dinner, or between meals: eating becomes a way of compensation for not smoking.

There are some studies, none definitive, that indicate that nicotine may have a fat-inhibiting action internally. Furthermore, heavy smoking dulls the sense of taste. The person who wakes up to full flavor after he or she stops smoking is likely to eat more food—perhaps without being aware of it.

As noted, some people are able to quit "cold turkey," stamping out that last cigarette and giving it up for good. Others succeed by switching first to low nicotine and tar cigarettes, which are considered less harmful generally. Then they cut down to fewer cigarettes per day, and fewer puffs per cigarette, not inhaling the smoke deeply. Some have given up smoking by joining group programs and using special devices, medication, and hypnosis.

If you have withdrawal symptoms, your physician probably can be helpful, perhaps advising certain medications to fit your personal needs. Good luck—and healthy, happy nonsmoking to you.

TO YOUR HEALTHIER, HAPPIER, LONGER LIFE . . .

Our total concern throughout this book has been to help you reduce pleasantly and healthfully to your desired weight, and then to stay trim thereafter. As an intelligent individual, you know the health and longevity benefits of not carrying the burden of excess weight. The health advantages are firmly established. Leanness is clearly an important factor in the increasing life expectancy in America—up from about forty-seven years in 1900 to seventy-three years and over today.

We recommend three fundamentals to help you stay in good health (not necessarily in this order):

1. Be trim . . .
2. Be active . . .
3. Get preventive medical checkups regularly, and seek immediate professional attention if any illness or health problem arises.

We have created Delicious Quick-Trim Diets and D.D. Nutri-Maintenance Eating as new, better ways of reducing and eating that you can live with and enjoy—for the rest of "your more attractive, healthier, longer life." As we have emphasized repeatedly, the doing is up to you.

Our heartfelt best wishes go with you. . . .

Samm Sinclair Baker

Sylvia Schur

INDEX

303

Chinese egg drop soup, D.D.
quick, 83–84
consommé Madrilène, D.D., 83
curried rice, D.D., 99
D.D., 134
gazpacho, D.D., 82
Hollandaise sauce, D.D., 141
mushroom soup epicure, D.D.,
83
with watercress, D.D., 84
vegetable, D.D., 68, 133–34, 148
brown rice cooked in, D.D., 98
curried tuna bisque, D.D., 81
dill salad dressing, D.D., 140
easy clam chowder with vegetables, D.D., 81
French salad dressing, D.D., 139
herbed vegetable juice cocktail,
D.D., 120
Italian salad dressing, D.D., 139
non-oil salad dressing, D.D., 140
see also Soup(s)
Brussels sprouts, 269
Buchwald, Art, 29
Bulimia, 297
Butter, 16, 52, 53, 60, 71, 148, 160,
177, 179, 185, 206, 236, 268, 269,
273, 295
Hollandaise sauce, D.D., 141

Cabbage, 146, 205, 269
garden veggie slaw, D.D., 197
health salad, D.D., 101
red and white coleslaw, D.D., 102
Caesar salad Roma, D.D., 101
Caffeine, 55, 59, 292–94
Cakes, 148
Calcium, 17, 251, 283, 290
Calisthenics, 156, 217
Calories, 14, 51–52, 177
burned during exercise, 211
chart, 219–21
in butter versus margarine, 251–52
in carbohydrates, fats, and proteins, 15–17, 19–20, 242–43
in cookbook and magazine recipes,
186–87
on Delicious Quick-Trim Diet, 19–
20, 21, 49–50, 51, 187
on Delicious Three-Day Vegetable
Diet, 145, 148
food contents checklist, 224–41

using, to maintain desired
weight, 181–83
intake versus expenditure, 14, 17,
144, 177, 221, 243, 252
laboratory measurement of, in food,
253
to maintain your desired weight,
181–83
typical day of Delicious Diet
Nutri-Maintenance Eating,
184–86
weight/calories chart, 183
in sweeteners, 251, 287–88
tradeoff system, 178
in typical American diet, 19–20
see also individual foods and types of
foods, e.g. Breads; Vegetable(s)
Cancer, 169, 277–79, 280, 298
Candies, 148, 239, 268–69, 288
Canoeing, 218
Cantaloupe, 291
slush, D.D., 112
Capers, 202
Cappucino, D.D. slim, 119
Caraway seeds, 202, 263
cottage cheese, D.D., 137
Carbohydrates, 15, 16–17, 242–43, 251,
281, 287
complex, 251, 281, 288
on D.D., 17, 19–20
facts about, 16–17
food contents checklist, 224–41
in typical American diet, 18, 19–20
Carlyle, Thomas, 36
Carrot(s), 146, 269, 291
and celery, D.D. julienne, 94
crudités with salsa dip, D.D., 122
fish fillet and, in lettuce wrap, D.D.
poached, 86–87
health salad, D.D., 101
salad, D.D., 100
steamed vegetable platter, D.D., 98
and turnip, D.D. puree of, 94–95
Case histories, 11–12, 127–28
Castelli, Dr. William, 39, 290
Cauliflower, 146, 269
Cayenne, 203, 263
Celery, 146, 269
carrots and, D.D. julienne, 94
crudités with salsa dip, D.D., 122
green beans and, D.D., 96
Celery seed, 203
Cellulite, 255

313

314

319

Tomato(es), sauce (*Continued*)
  seafood Seviche, D.D., 194
  soup, D.D. chicken-vegetable, 80
  vegetable mélange in foil, D.D.,
    96
Tooth decay, 287
Toward the Conquest of Cancer (Beattie),
  279
Tradeoff system, 178
Travel, 174, 295–97
Triglycerides, 280–81
Troisgros, Jean, 201
Troisgros, Pierre, 201
Trout, herb grilled, 86
Tumeric, 204
Tuna:
  apple salad with greens, D.D., 103
  bisque, D.D. curried, 81
  canned, 52, 291
  mushroom salad, D.D., 104
  spicy seafood salad, D.D., 108
Turkey, 53, 163, 177
  breast baked with tarragon and
    white wine, D.D., 91
  checklist of herbs, spices, and sea-
    sonings for, 203
  cooking methods for, 53
  gingered stir-fry vegetables with,
    D.D., 88
  removing skin and visible fat from,
    53, 177
  salad with green grapes, D.D. cur-
    ried, 105
  scaloppine alla Marsala, 129
  steaks Forestière, D.D., 197–98
Turnip(s), 146, 269
  carrot and, D.D. puree of, 94–95

Uncoffee au lait, D.D., 119
U.S. Department of Agriculture, 223,
  241, 281
University of Texas Medical Branch,
  290
Upton, Dr. Arthur, 279

Vacations, 174, 295–97
Variety Diet, *see* Delicious Variety
  (With Meat) Quick-Trim Diet
Veal, 204
  burgers, 204
  D.D. lean, 129–30

cooking methods for, 205
kebabs with onions, pepper
  squares, and mushrooms,
  D.D., 130
scalloppine alla Marsala, 129
Vegetable(s), 11, 92–98, 161, 164, 169,
  180, 250, 282, 283, 287, 291, 292,
  296
  broth, D.D., 68, 133–34, 148
  brown rice cooked in, D.D., 98
  curried tuna bisque, D.D., 81
  dill dressing, D.D., 140
  easy clam chowder with vege-
    tables, D.D., 81
  French salad dressing, D.D., 139
  herbed vegetable juice cocktail,
    D.D., 120
  Italian salad dressing, D.D., 139
  non-oil salad dressing, D.D., 140
  calorie content, 229–31, 269, 271–
    72
  checklist of herbs, spices, and sea-
    sonings for, 203–204
  creativity in preparing and serving,
    207–208
  food contents checklist, 229–31
  frozen, 271
  garden veggie slaw, D.D., 197
  mélange in foil, D.D., 96
  permitted on Delicious Quick-Trim
    Diet, 53
  permitted on Delicious Three-Day
    Vegetable Diet, 146
  as protein source, 10
  shopping tips, 51, 60–61
  as snacks, 69, 207
    crudités with salsa dip, D.D., 122
    zucchini sticks with herb dip,
      D.D., 122
  soups:
    chicken-, tomato, D.D., 80
    easy clam chowder with, D.D.,
      81
    gazpacho, D.D., 82
  specialité with zesty broccoli, D.D.,
    107
  steamed platter, D.D., 98
  stir-fry:
    with chicken or turkey, D.D. gin-
      gered, 88
    and rice salad with water chest-
      nuts, D.D., 103
  variety of, 207, 269

320

ACKNOWLEDGMENTS

My warmest thanks to wife Natalie for her indispensable contributions to this book and always to our family, Jeff and Ester, Wendy and Bob, for most helpful and supportive reading and comments, and to Michael and Caleb, for being.

To Stanley for expert attention and concern now and through the years.

To Perry for knowing guidance and steadfast endeavor.

To Marc for his intelligence, decency, and friendship.

S.S.B.

My appreciation and warm thanks for husband Saul's interest in tasting, honesty in evaluation, and confirming loss of pounds in the process! Professional and personal thanks to my associates at Creative Food Service—Judith Gorfain, Tracy Duckworth-Spak, Diane Farewell-Walsh, Pam Dukas, Lillie Charlton, and Patricia Shoemaker—for their intelligent and responsive participation in manuscript processing and checking, calorie calculations, and recipe testing.

S.Z.S.

Samm Sinclair Baker, who has been called by *The New York Times* America's leading self-help author, has written 28 popular books to date, including the six hugely successful diet books he wrote with two late and legendary diet doctors, Irwin Stillman and Herman Tarnower. He lives in Westchester County with his wife, Natalie, who is a professional artist, art teacher, and coauthor with him on the popular artbook *Family Treasury of Art*. They have two grown children, both doctors.

Sylvia Schur has been a food editor of leading national magazines, including *Seventeen* and *Parade*, and is also a noted food writer, with more than a dozen cookbooks to her credit. Currently she is a food consultant to a number of leading companies, and is the founder/director of Creative Food Service in New Rochelle, New York. Mrs. Schur lives in Westchester County with her husband, Saul, and is visited from time to time by their three grown children and their families.